Vorwort

Hallo lieber Leser, hallo liebe Leserin,

dieser erste von insgesamt 4 Bänden vermittelt Ihnen das komplette theoretische Wissen sowie die wichtigsten Basistechniken des kinesiologischen Tapens.

Dieses Wissen ist Ihr Rüstzeug für alle weiteren Techniken und Anwendungen, die Sie – gepaart mit dem einzigartigen Lernkonzept – ganz intuitiv werden erlernen können.

„Einfach und effektiv“

Sie erhalten einen umfangreichen Überblick über alle Techniken, die sich bis heute am Besten in der Praxis bewährt haben, inklusive Methoden aus Japan und Südkorea. Darüber hinaus verrate ich Ihnen viele Tricks und Kniffe, mit denen Sie ganz besonders gute Erfolge erzielen können sowie Anwendungen bei Indikationen, die viele Therapeuten bis heute nicht kennen. Somit erhalten Sie einen Vorsprung durch Wissen.

Ich werde Ihnen anhand von Anwendungsbildern zeigen, wie das kinesiologische Tapen ursprünglich gedacht war.

Zum Erlernen des gesamten Basiswissens ist dies der wichtigste Band!

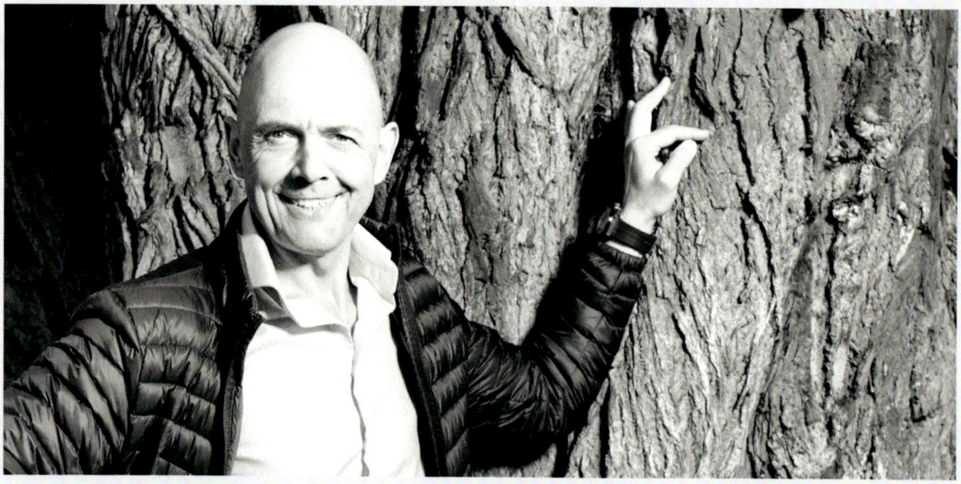

Olaf Kandt, kinesiologischer Experte

Preface

Dear reader,

This, the first of four volumes, provides you with all the theoretical knowledge and the most important basic kinesiology taping techniques. This knowledge will give you the tools you need for all the other techniques and methods.

With my unique approach anyone can learn taping techniques intuitively.

"Easy and effective"

This volume gives an extensive overview of all the techniques that have proven themselves in practice including methods from Japan and South Korea. You will find many tips and tricks which will help you in achieving exceedingly good results along with techniques for indications not many therapists know about.

The knowledge I share with you will therefore give you the edge.

I will show you how kinesiology taping was originally conceived.

This is the most important volume for learning all of the basic knowledge.

Der Autor Olaf Kandt

Jahrgang 1964, Medical Trainer

Seit 1992 trainiert und berät er Ärzte, Pflegepersonal, Physiotherapeuten und Heilpraktiker in Kliniken, Arztpraxen, sportphysiotherapeutischen Einrichtungen und Schulen sowie Therapeuten aus dem Profisport. Olaf Kandt ist weltweit als Trainer und Berater tätig. Zudem betreut er als Consulter einen internationalen medizinischen Konzern.

Schwerpunkte seiner Arbeit sind die Themen der modernen funktionellen Behandlungsmethoden im Sport-, Praxis- und Klinikbereich. In den letzten 20 Jahren hat Olaf sich zum Spezialisten für kinesiologische Tapetechniken, klassisches Tapen, Gips- und Castanwendungen, Kompressionverbände und frühfunktionelle Versorgungstechniken bei Sportverletzungen entwickelt.

Sein Erfolg basiert auf langjähriger Erfahrung im Umgang mit den unterschiedlichsten Kundengruppen. Olaf Kandt hat sich in zahlreichen Seminaren ein umfangreiches Wissen in den Bereichen Rhetorik, Verkaufspsychologie und Präsentationstechniken angeeignet. Er bereichert seine Fortbildungen mit lebendigen Tipps und Tricks, die in der Praxis leicht umsetzbar sind und so zu einem schnellen Erfolg bei den Teilnehmern führen.

Alle Seminare, Kongresse und Workshops sind lernphysiologisch sehr abwechslungsreich aufgebaut. Die aktive Mitarbeit aller Teilnehmer beim Anwenden und Üben des Gelernten ist ein weiterer Baustein des Erfolgs.

Olaf Kandt ist zudem verantwortlicher Berater bei Produktentwicklungen für Medical Produkte.

Werdegang

- Ausbildung zum examinierten Krankenpfleger, Schwerpunkt Sporttraumatologie, Sportphysiotherapie und Unfallchirurgie

- Leiter der Medical Trainer
  Beiersdorf & BSN medical in Hamburg

- Geschäftsführer seiner Firma
  OKAMED Medizinproduktevertrieb
  www.okamed.de / www.okamed.com

- Geschäftsführer seiner Trainingsacademy **Olaf Kandt international medical academy**
  www.ok-academy.com

Konzeption und Durchführung von Fortbildungsveranstaltungen und Trainings zur Ausbildung der nationalen Anwendungsberater und der Topkunden im In- und Ausland (Kliniken, Therapeuten im Profisport z.B. Bundesliga und Nationalmannschaften).

Seit 2006 ist er selbständiger Medical Trainer weltweit.

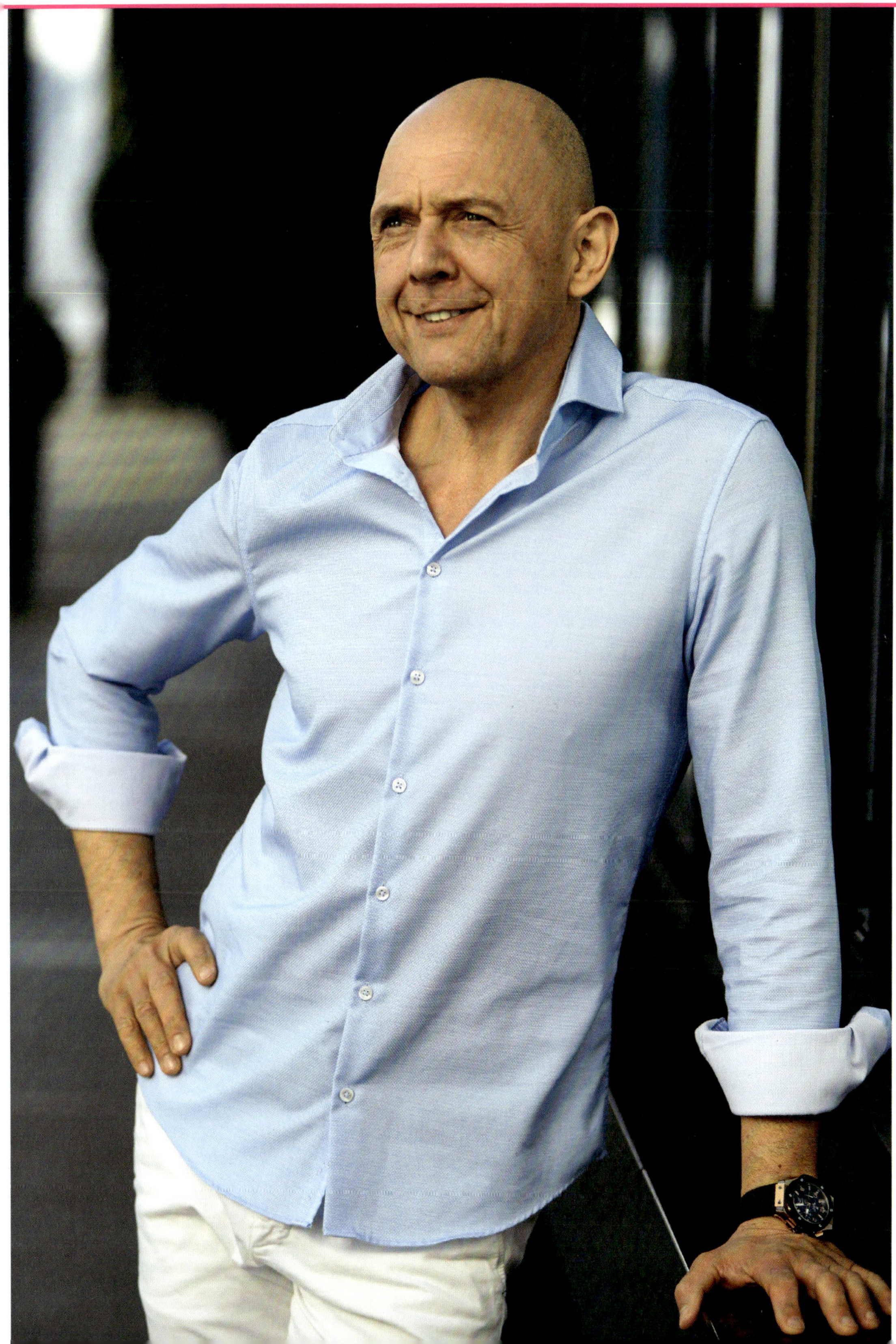

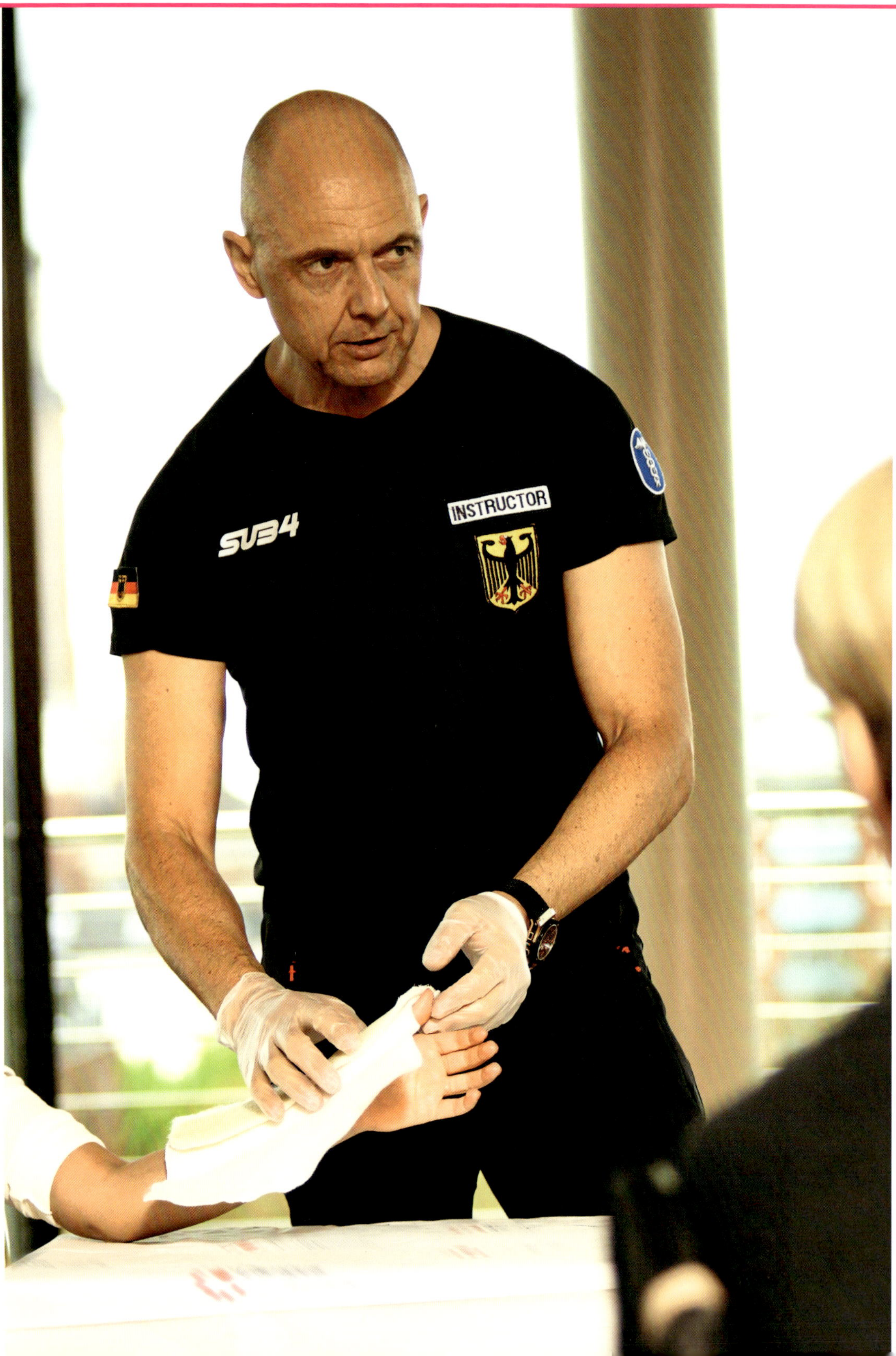
INSTRUCTOR
SUB4

The author Olaf Kandt

Born in 1964, medical trainer

Since 1992 has trained and advised doctors, nurses, physiotherapists and non-medical practitioners in hospitals, medical practices, sports physiotherapy establishments and schools as well as therapists working in professional sport. Olaf Kandt works as a trainer and consultant all over the world. In addition, he acts as a consultant to an international medical concern.

In his work, he specialises in modern functional treatment methods in sport, medical practices and the hospital setting. Over the last 20 years, Olaf has become an expert in kinesiology taping techniques, classic taping, the use of plaster and casts, compression dressings and early functional treatment techniques for sports injuries.

His success is based on many years' experience dealing with a wide range of client groups. Olaf Kandt has attended numerous seminars, acquiring extensive knowledge in the fields of rhetoric, sales psychology and presentation techniques. He enriches his training courses with lively tips and tricks that are easy to implement in practice and quickly enable the participants to achieve successful outcomes.

All seminars, conferences and workshops are designed to be very varied, with the physiology of learning in mind. Actively involving all participants in applying and practising what they have learned is a further factor in his success.

Furthermore, Olaf Kandt is a consultant on product developments for medical devices.

Career

- Trained as a registered nurse specialising in sports trauma, sports physiotherapy and accident surgery
- Director of Medical Trainer Beiersdorf & BSN medical in Hamburg
- Managing Director of his company **OKAMED** GmbH
- Managing Director of his Academy for Trainings: **Olaf Kandt international medical academy**
  www.ok-academy.com

Design and implementation of continuing professional development events and courses to train national application consultants and top customers in Germany and internationally (hospitals, therapists working in professional sport, e.g. the German Bundesliga and national teams).

Olaf Kandt has been a freelance medical trainer since 2006 and works all over the world.

Das Olaf-Kandt-Lernkonzept

Das Geheimnis meines Erfolges, meiner Lernmethode und meines Fortbildungskonzeptes seit mehr als 20 Jahren.

Ich habe bereits erfolgreich zwei Bücher über die Anwendung von Gitterpflastern veröffentlicht. Durch die bildreiche Darstellung der Anwendungen ist es simpel und dennoch einzigartig. Die Leser und Anwender sind begeistert.

Das Besondere

Ich schreibe meine Bücher so, wie ich sie selbst gerne als tägliches Werkzeug in der Anwendung benutzen möchte.

- Schnell zu den praktischen Übungen.
- Mit wenig Text und vielen Bildern die Techniken erlernen.

Wenig Text

Niemand liest gerne lange Texte, wenn er ein Anwendungsbuch für den täglichen Einsatz sucht. Die Theorie soll kurz und knapp sein, nur das Wichtigste genannt werden.

Viele Tipps

Sollte es mal nicht gleich klappen, nicht entmutigen lassen, ich gebe Ihnen Tipps und zeige Alternativen auf.

Im Praxisteil

Viele Bilder zeigen Ihnen wie es geht, somit können Sie direkt starten.

Meine Kurse

Sie können mich jederzeit buchen. Nach Terminabsprache komme ich gern in Ihre Räumlichkeiten.

Schreiben Sie mir einfach eine E-Mail:
info@okamed.de

Oder besuchen Sie meine Seite
www.okamed.de

Oder folgen Sie mir auf Facebook:
Olaf Kandt Fortbildungen

So macht Lernen Spaß!

The Olaf-Kandt-Learning concept

The secret to my success, my teaching method and my training approach for over 20 years.

I have already successfully published two books about the use of cross-tapes. Their liberal use of pictures makes them easy to use and yet unique. Readers and users are thrilled.

What makes my approach special

I write my books in the way I myself would like to be able to use them as a daily tool.

- They get quickly to the practical exercises.
- They teach the techniques using little text and lots of pictures.

Little text

Nobody like to read long texts when looking for a practical book for everyday use. The theory should be short and sweet, explaining only the most important information.

Lots of tips

Should something not work immediately, do not be discouraged. I will give you tips and show you alternatives.

The practical section

There is a large number of pictures showing you what to do so that you can get started straightaway.

My courses

You can book me anytime. I will gladly visit you at your premises, by prior arrangement.

Simply e-mail me at:
info@okamed.com

Or visit my website
www.okamed.com

Or follow me on Facebook:
Olaf Kandt Training Courses

Making learning fun!

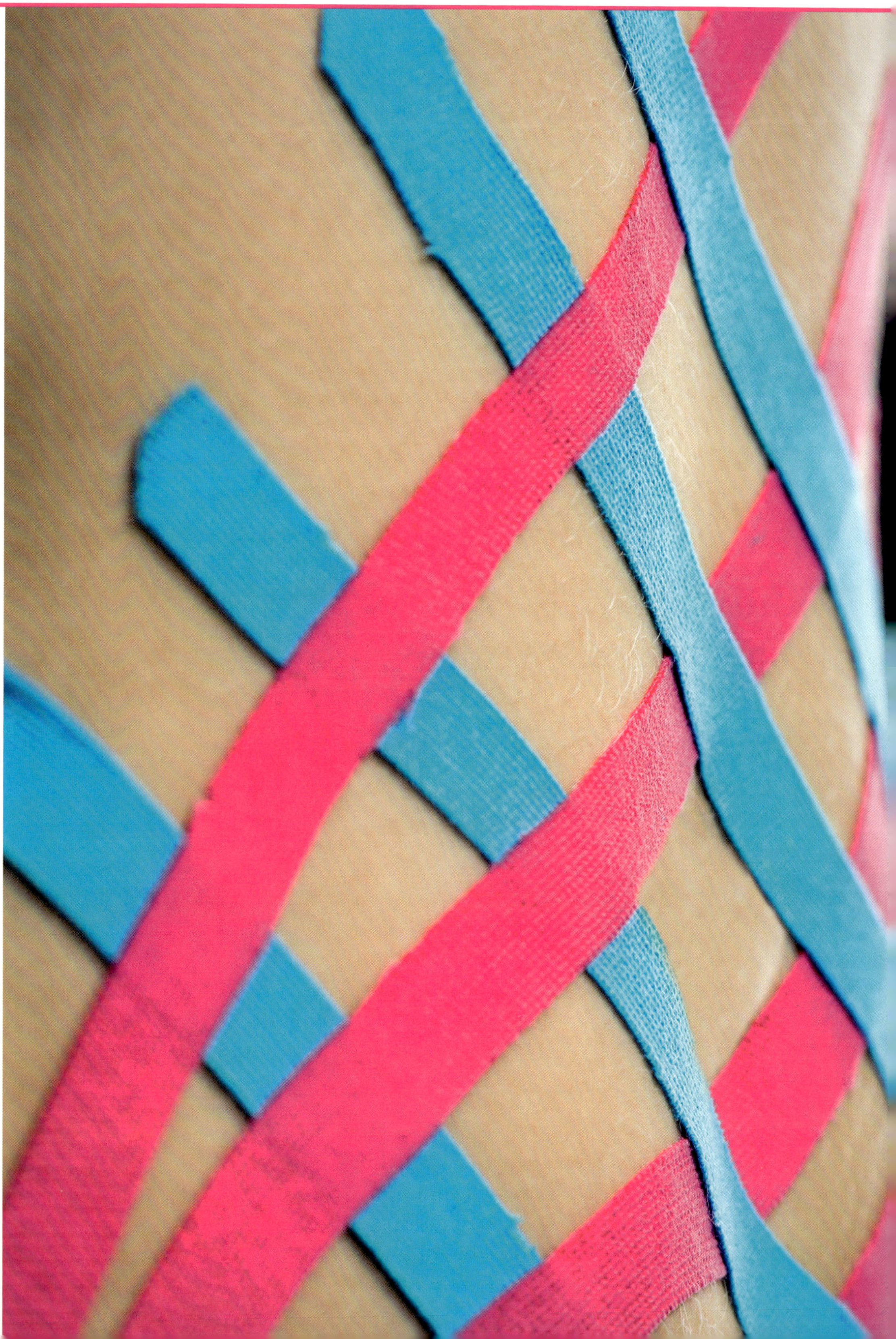

Die Idee
The Idea

Über die Hautoberfläche alle darunter liegenden Strukturen beeinflussen.

(Muskeln, Sehnen, Bänder, Nerven, Lymphgefäße, Rezeptoren)

Affect all underlying structures via the skinsurface.

(Muscles, tendons, ligaments, nerves, lymphatic vessels, receptors)

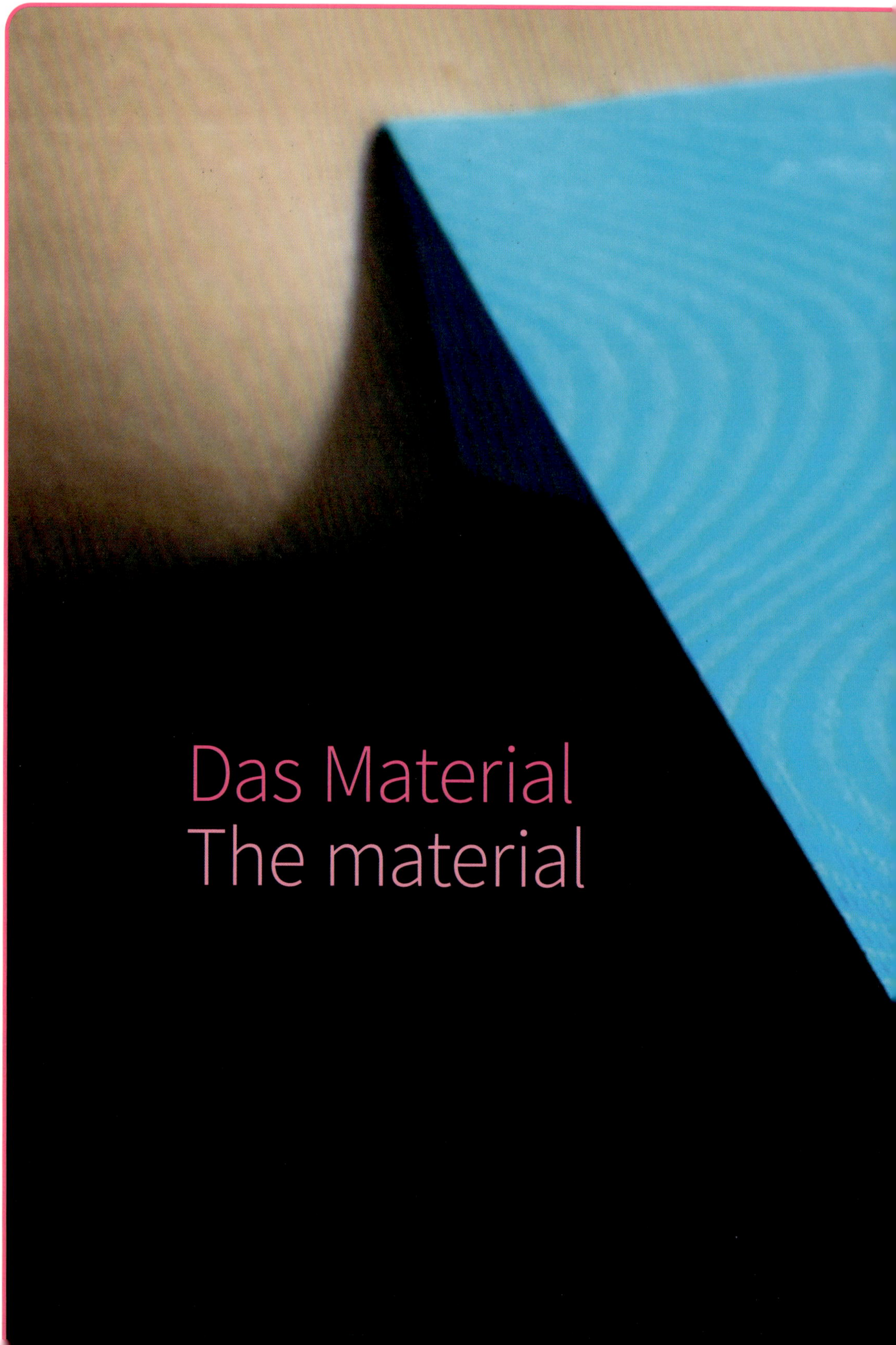

Das Material
The material

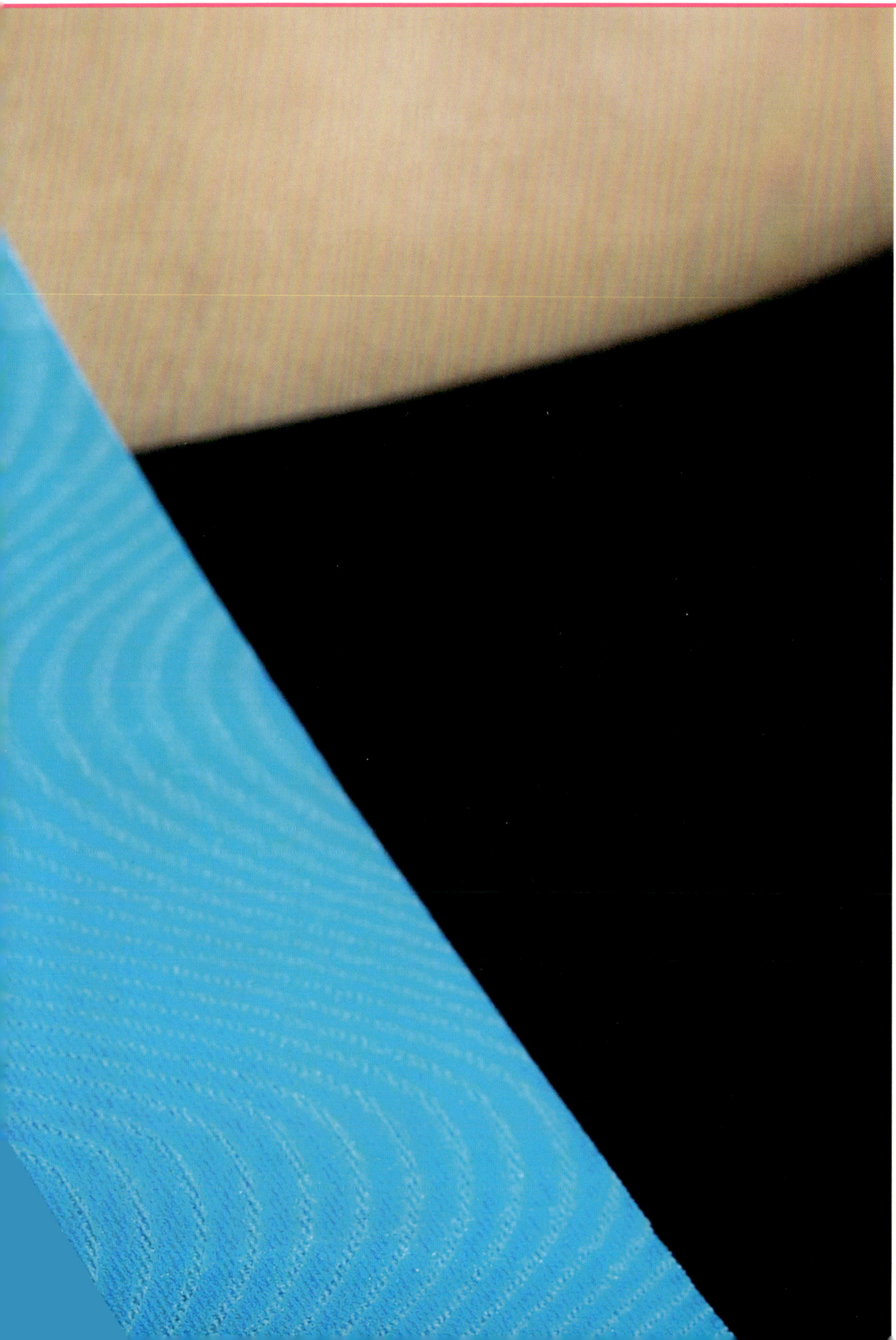

Das Material der Tapes

Das Tape besteht aus einem Baumwollgewebe mit einem hautfreundlichen Polyacrylatkleber.

Der Kleber ist in einer sinusförmigen Wellenform aufgetragen. Dies ermöglicht ein Ablaufen von Flüssigkeit und sichert so die Klebkraft auch beim Duschen oder Baden.

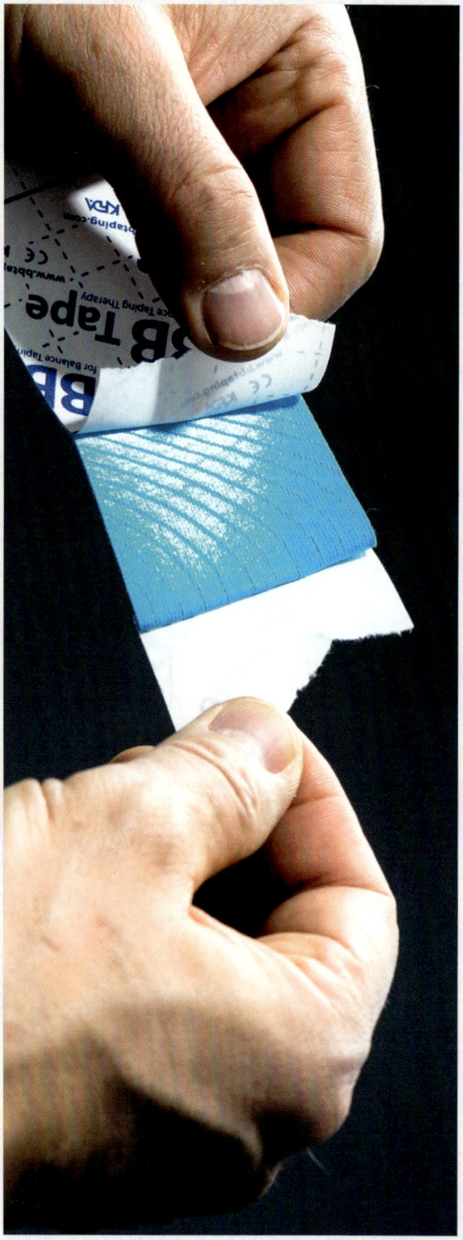

Die Farben und Drucke

Die Tapes sind in verschiedenen Farben und Mustern erhältlich. Auf Material und Wirkungsweise hat das jedoch keinen Einfluss. Farben und Muster haben lediglich modischen Charakter.

Die Wirkung der Farbe auf den Menschen

Etwas, das wir als schön empfinden, kann zu mehr Wohlempfinden und damit Therapietoleranz führen. Es ist daher ratsam, dem Patienten eine Auswahl an Farben und Mustern anzubieten, so dass er wie bei einem Kleidungsstück das für ihn passende wählen kann.

The tape material

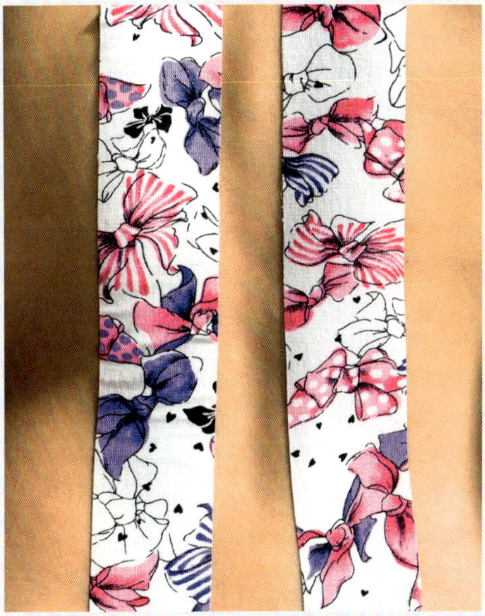

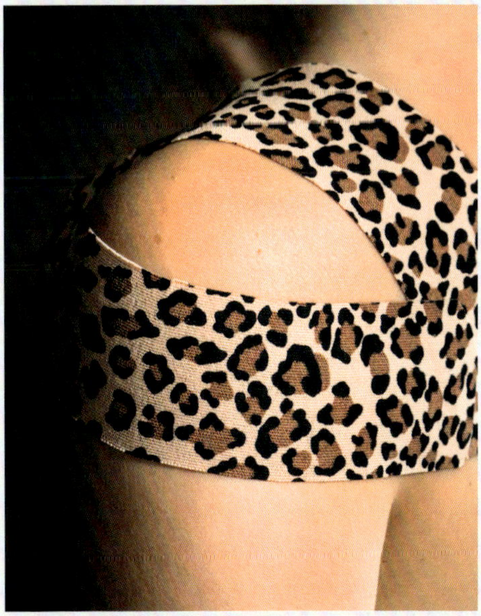

The tape is made of cotton with a skin-friendly acrylic adhesive.

The adhesive is applied in a sine wave pattern. This allows fluid to drain and therefore ensures proper adhesion while showering or bathing.

The colours and prints

Tapes with prints are very popular.

The colour

Tapes are available in various colours, although these have no effect on performance.

The effect of colour on people

The colour is merely a fashion statement, but choosing a favourite colour might increase the patient's therapy adherence.

Therefore I advise you to offer patients a range of colours or tapes with prints. Anything considered attractive may result in better well-being.

Die Wirkung
The effect

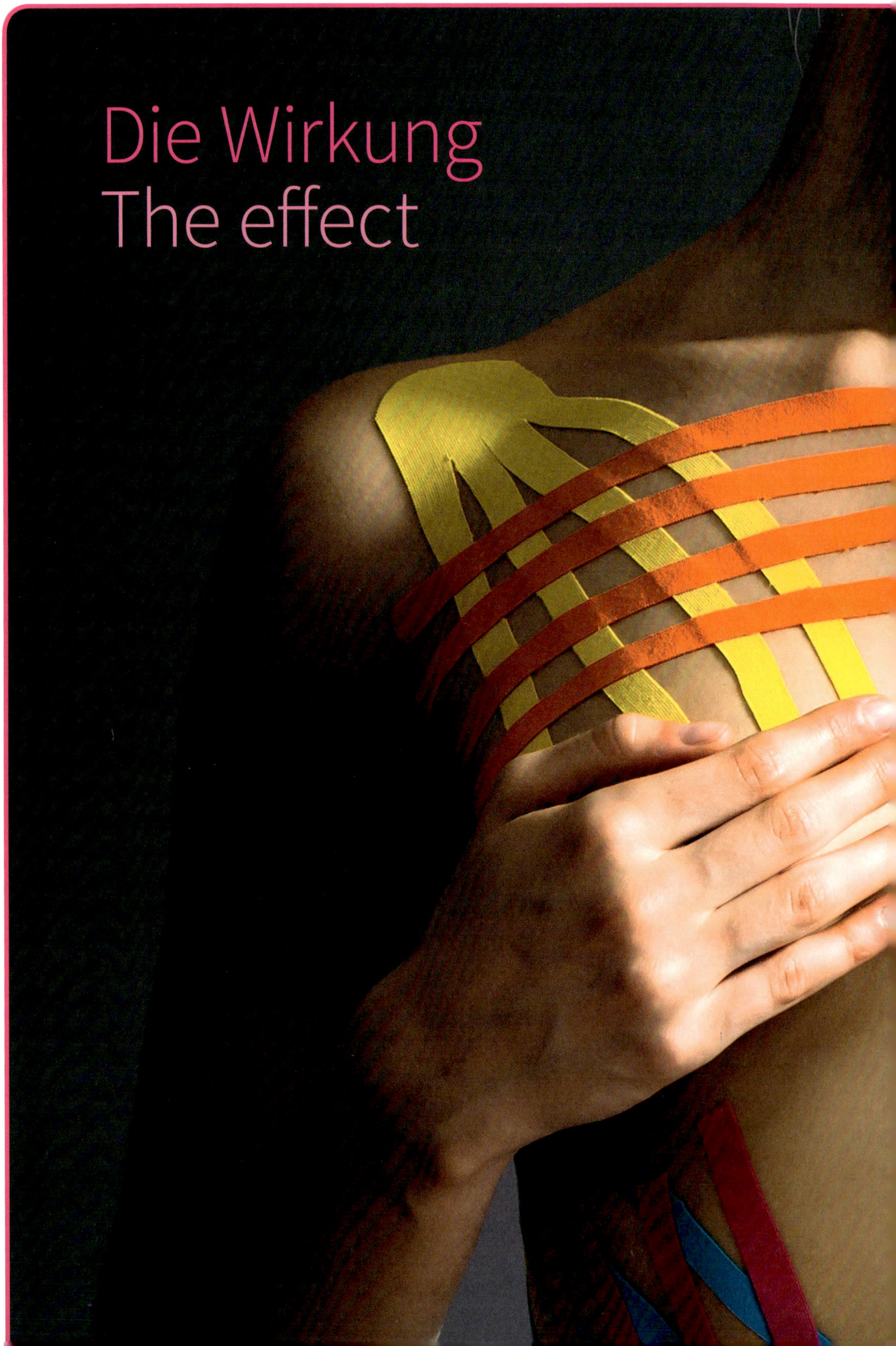

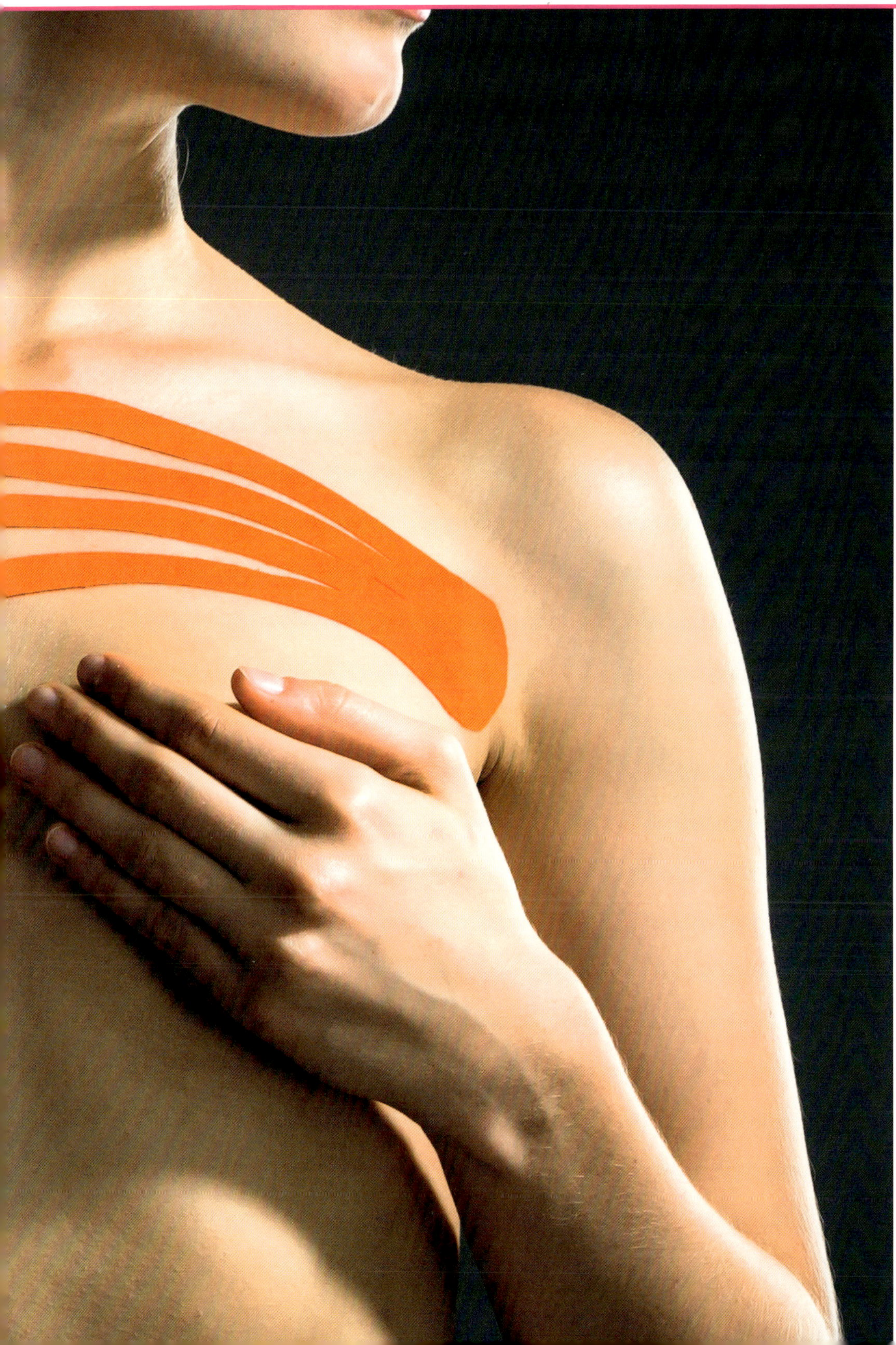

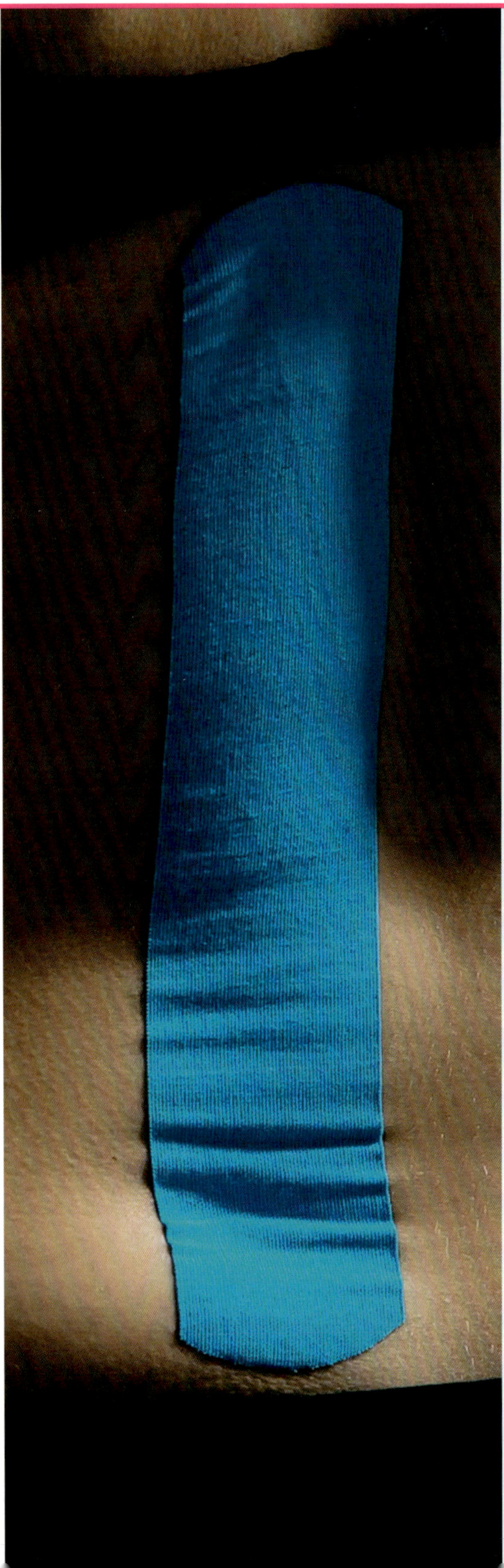

Entlastung der Hautoberfläche

Während der gesamten Tragezeit des Tapes wird die Hautoberfläche konstant angehoben. Dies erzeugt kontinuierliche Entlastungsreize.

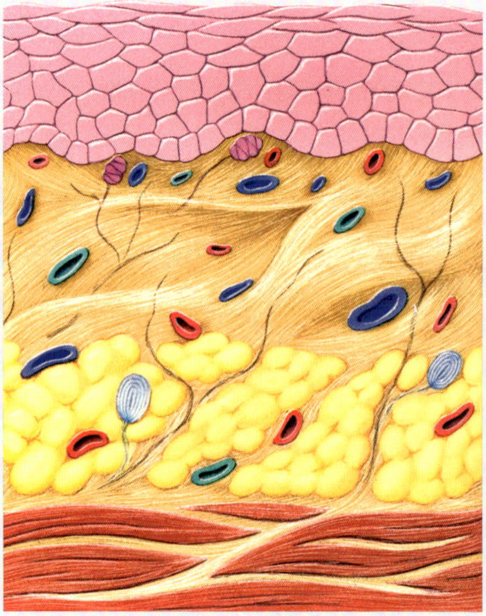

Quelle: BSN medical GmbH

Ohne Tape | Without tape

Durch Hautanhebung werden alle Hautrezeptoren aktiviert sowie die Lymph- und Kapillargefäße gedehnt.

Dadurch wird der Stoffwechsel im Gewebe erhöht, alle Strukturen werden wieder besser versorgt. Muskeln können wieder besser arbeiten, Entzündungen besser und schneller abheilen.

Decompression of the skin

While the tape is worn, the surface of the skin is being constantly lifted the whole time. This creates continuous decompression stimuli.

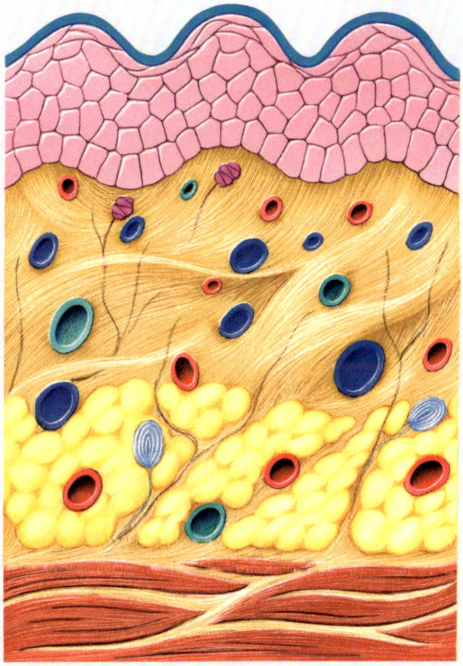

Quelle: BSN medical GmbH

Mit Tape | With tape

The skin-lifting effect activates all of the skin's receptors and stretches the lymphatic vessels and capillaries.

This increases the metabolism in the tissues, improving the perfusion of all structures. Muscles are able to work better again and inflammation heals better and more rapidly.

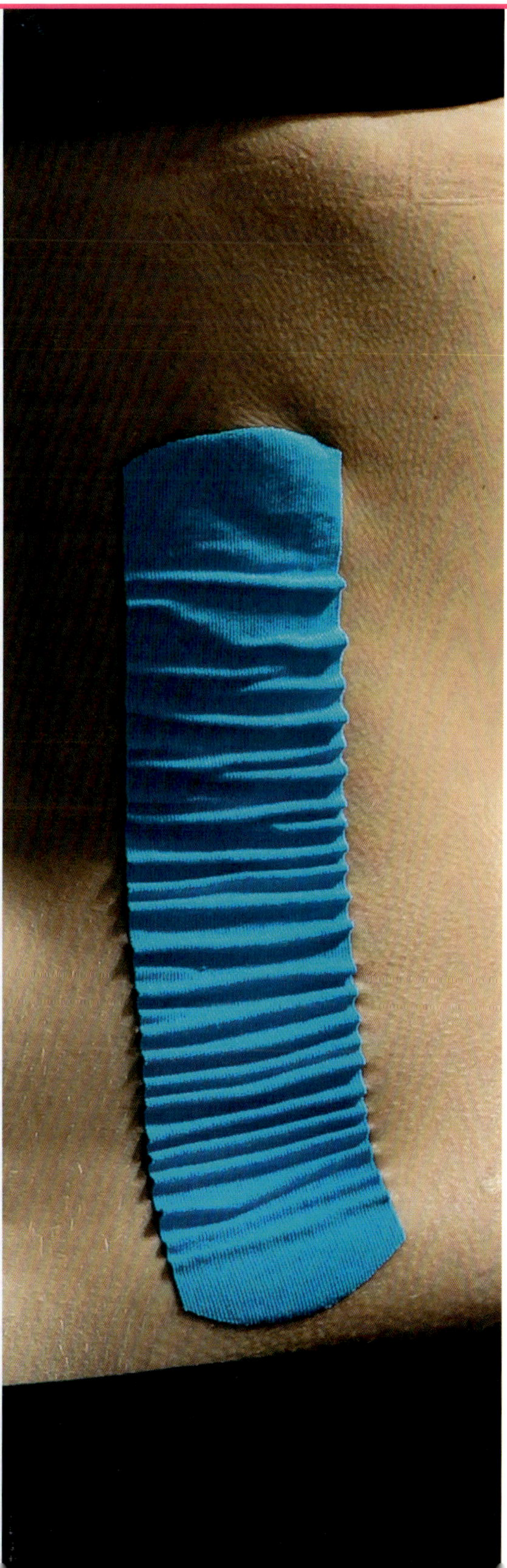

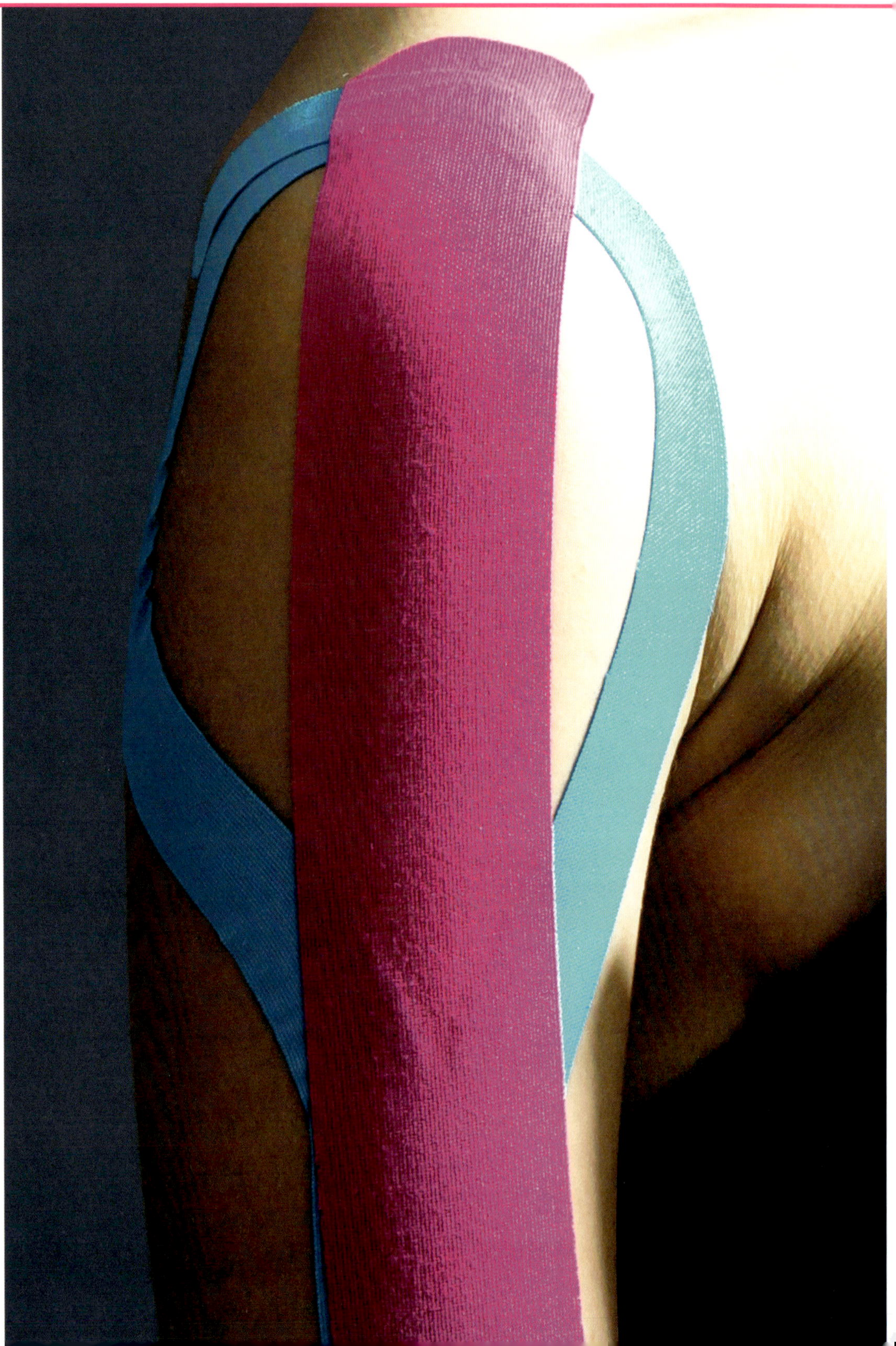

Spezielle Wirkung
Special effect

Stabilisierung von Gelenken (Sprunggelenk, Handgelenk, Schultergelenk etc.)

Die Reizung der Hautrezeptoren durch die elastischen Tapebänder führt zu einer effektiven Stabilisierung der Gelenke, ohne diese in der Beweglichkeit zu blockieren.

Korrektur von Fehlstellungen (Haltungskorrektur, Gelenkfehlstellungen wie z. B. Kniegelenk, Schultergelenk, Wirbelsäule, Fußfehlstellungen, etc.)

Durch gezieltes Aufbringen der Tapebänder mit dem angegebenen Zug kann effektiv auf Gelenkveränderungen Einfluss genommen werden.

Joint stabilisation (ankle, wrist, shoulder, etc.)

The stimulation of the skin's receptors by the elastic tape strips brings about effective joint stabilisation without blocking joint mobility.

Correction of misalignments (posture correction, joint misalignment, e.g. of the knee, shoulder, spine, foot, etc.)

Targeted application of tape strips with the stated stretch can have a real influence on joint changes.

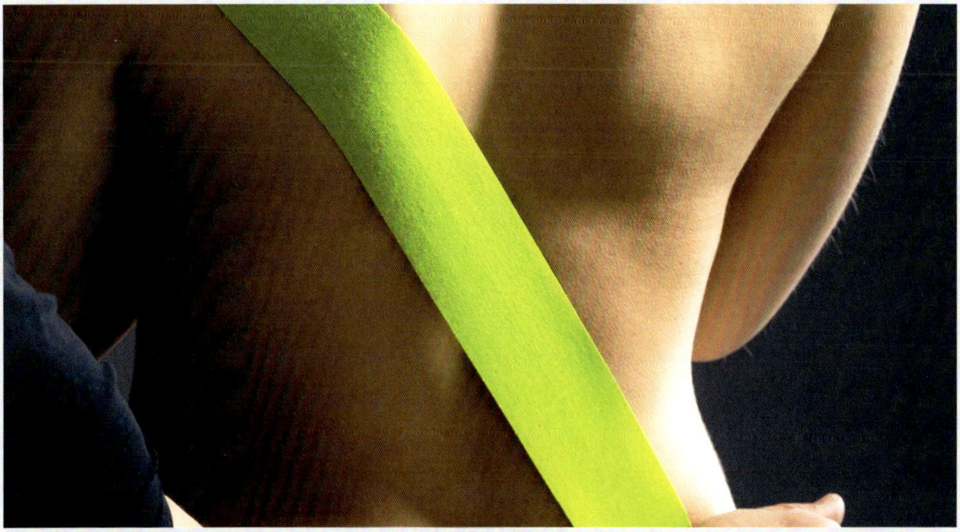

Effekt des Hautabhebereizes

Die Dehnung der Lymph- und Kapillargefäße führt zu einer Dehnung der Gefäßwände. Dadurch wird die Durchblutung gegsteigert. Zusätzlich kann eingelagerte Flüssigkeit im Gewebe schneller abtransportiert werden. Ein weiterer Effekt ist das Aktivieren aller Hautrezeptoren durch den Zugreiz der Tapebänder.

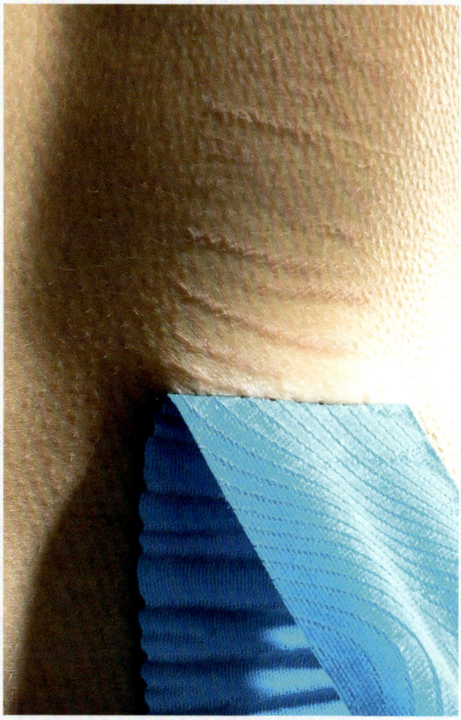

In der Folge werden Triggerpunkte, Reflexzonen und Akupunkturpunkte angesteuert und entlastet.

Effekt: Muskeln, Sehnen und Organe reagieren mit Entlastungsreizen. Der Stoffwechsel im Gewebe wird aktiviert

Ergebnisse

- Ödeme werden reduziert
- Hämatome werden sehr schnell resorbiert
- Ödemneigungen, z. B. nach einer Operation, werden reduziert, Hämatome sehr schnell abgebaut
- Der Stoffwechsel im verletzen Areal wird verbessert
- Schmerzen werden reduziert
- Schnellere Heilung möglich
- Bessere Mobilisierung

Effect of the skin-lifting stimulus

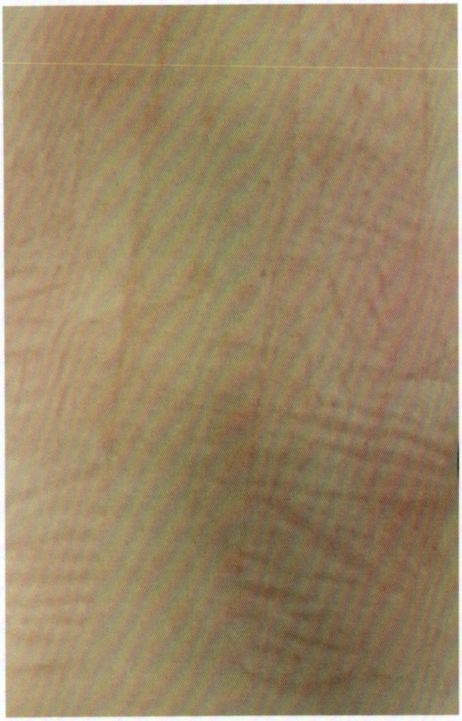

Stretching the lymphatic vessels and capillaries ensures much better drainage of stored fluid. At the same time, the receptors underneath the skin respond to the stretch stimulus. Furthermore, all cutaneous receptors will be activated through the tension of the tapes.

As a result, trigger points, reflex zones and acupuncture points are activated and decompressed.

The effect: muscles, tendons and organs respond by decompressing. The metabolism in the tissues is activated.

The results

- Oedema is reduced
- Haematomas will be absorbed quickly
- Susceptibility to oedema, e.g. after surgery, is reduced and haematomas are broken down very rapidly
- Metabolism in the injured area is improved
- Pain is reduced
- More rapid healing is possible
- Mobilisation is better

Weitere Effekte

Bindegewebe (Faszien)

Verklebungen im gesamten Bindegewebe können mit Hilfe des Tapes gelöst werden. Dies führt zu einer gezielten Schmerzentlastung und sofortigen besseren Beweglichkeit.

Interessant für Patienten

- mit chronischer Bewegungseinschränkung an den Gelenken
- mit Schmerzen im Bindegewebe z. B. nach OP oder Trauma

Reflexzonen-System

Über die Entlastungsreize der Hautoberfläche kann gezielt auf alle Reflexzonen Einfluss genommen werden.

Einsatzmöglichkeiten

- Beeinflussung der inneren Organe
- Effektive Unterstützung vieler Therapiemethoden

Nerven

Auch das neurologische System kann durch die tapeinduzierten Reize beeinflusst werden.

Beispiele

- Spastiken
- Chronische Schmerzzustände (Ischias, Trigeminus, Karpaltunnelsyndrom)
- Schmerzhafte Schübe (Arthrose, Arthritis, Gicht, Rheuma, Parkinson, Multiple Sklerose)
- Kontrakturen
- Paresen (Apoplex, Fußhebeschwäche, Wahrnehmungsprobleme)
- Schlaganfall: Kann jede Therapie unterstützen

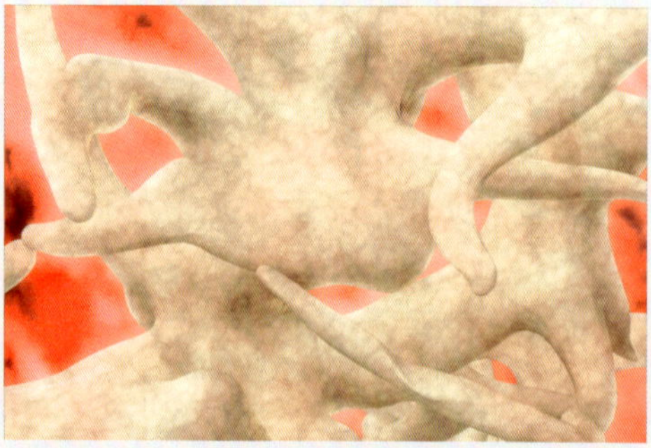

Further effects

Connective tissues (fascia)

Adhesions throughout the connective tissues can be released with the aid of the tape. This leads to targeted pain relief and immediately improved mobility.

Interesting for patients

- with chronic movement restriction at the joints
- with connective tissue pain, e.g. after surgery or trauma

Reflex zones

All reflex zones can be influenced specifically through the decompression stimuli at the skin's surface.

Potential uses

- To influence the internal organs
- To provide effective support for many treatment methods

Nerves

The neurological system can also be influenced by the tape-induced stimuli.

Examples

- Spasticity
- Chronic pain states (sciatic nerve, trigeminal nerve, carpal tunnel syndrome)
- Painful flares (arthrosis, arthritis, gout, rheumatism, Parkinson's disease, multiple sclerosis)
- Contractures
- Palsy (stroke, peroneal nerve injury, foot drop, perceptual problems)
- Stroke: Can support each kind of therapy.

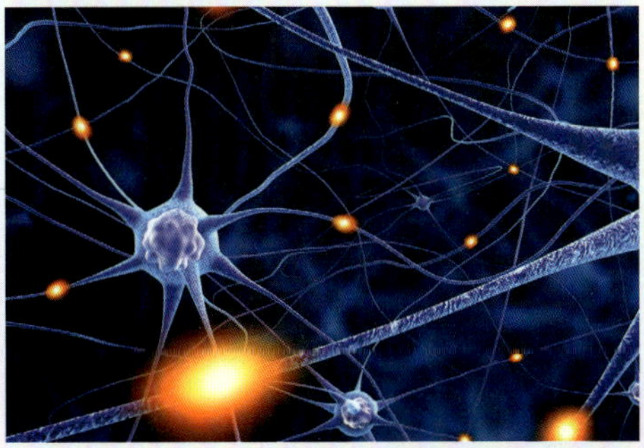

Die Anwendung
The application

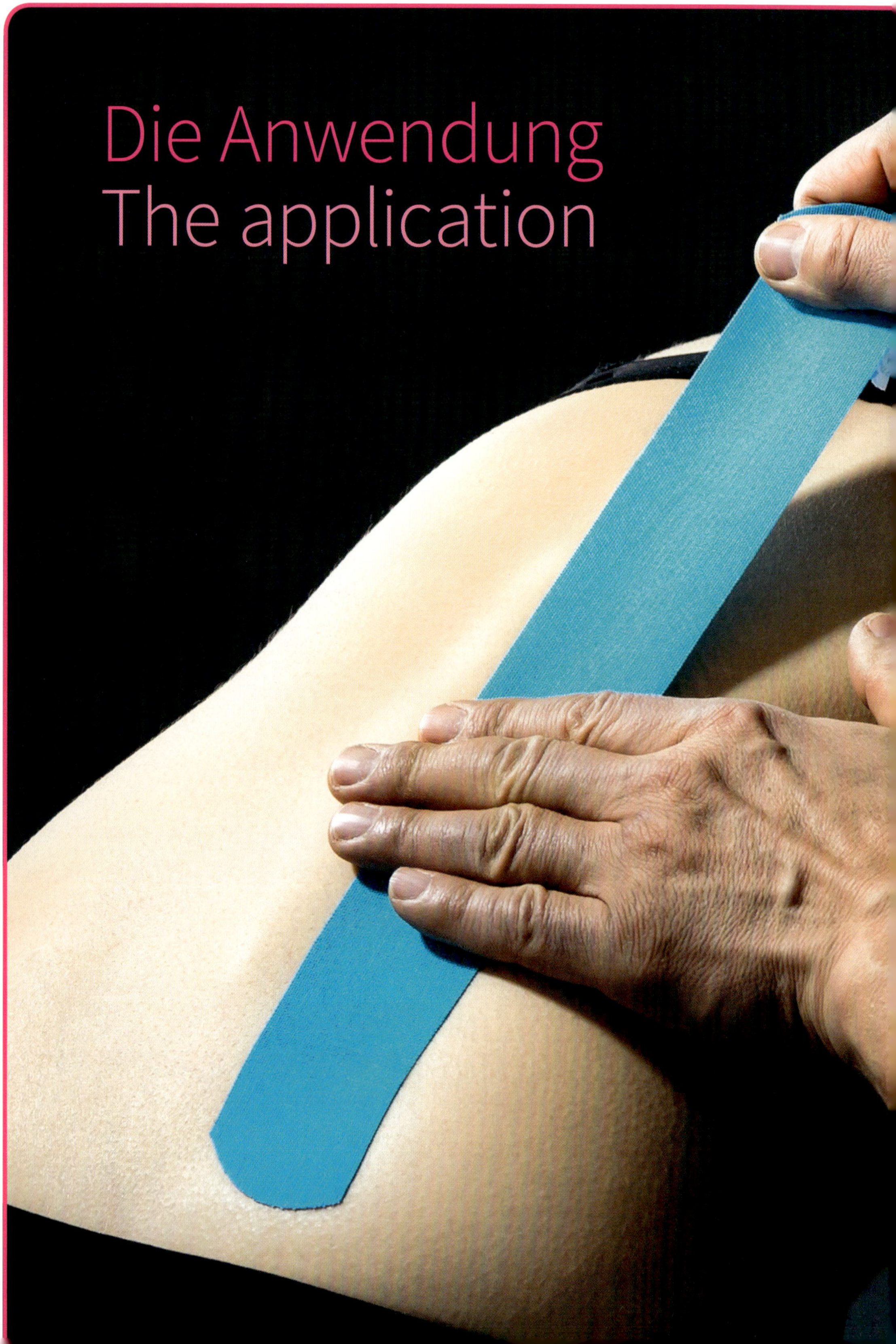

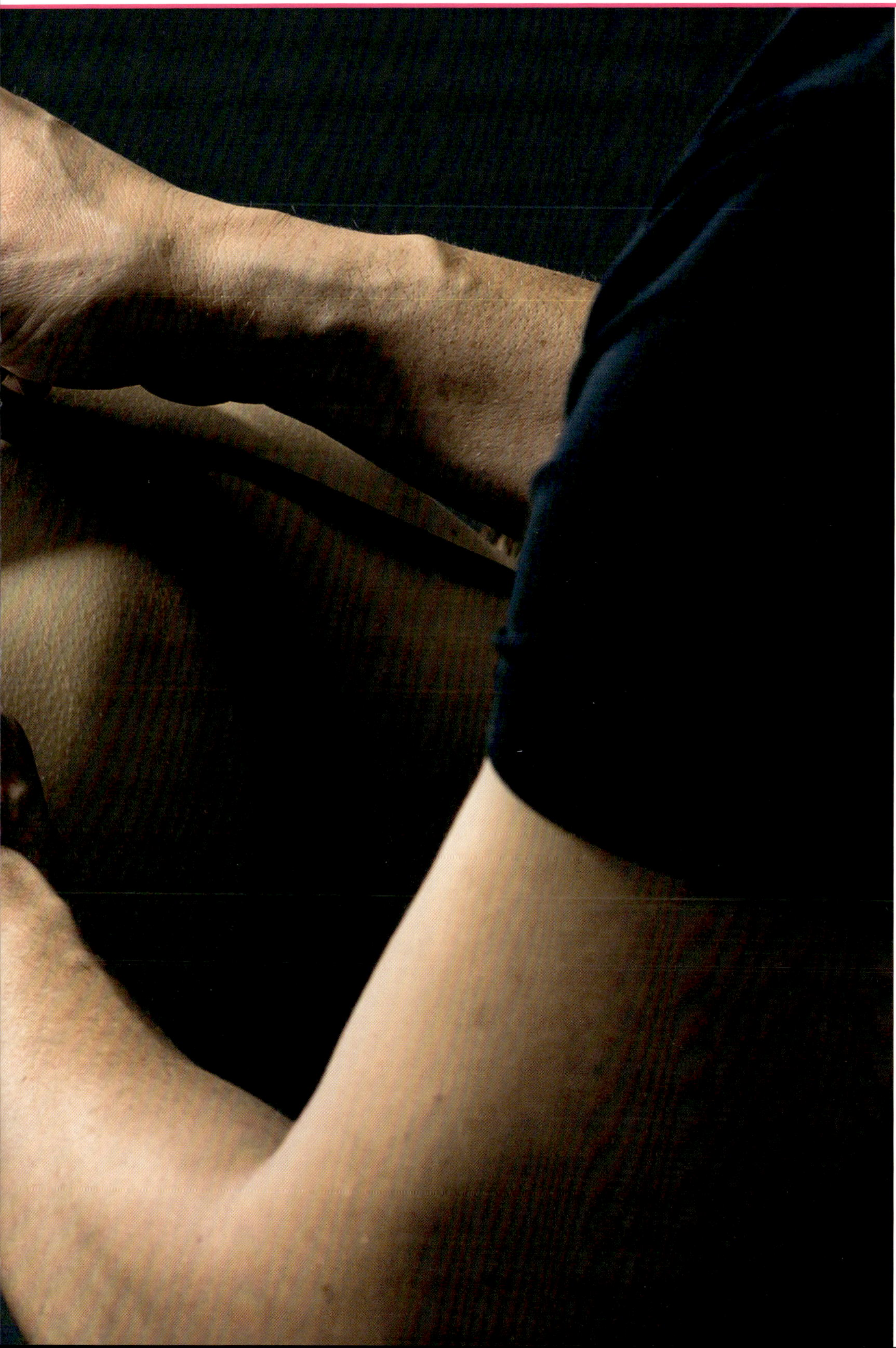

Vor dem Aufbringen

Bitte vor dem Anlegen der Tapebänder folgende Hinweise beachten:

- Die Haut muss trocken sein.
- Haare sollten entweder gekürzt oder abrasiert werden.
- Die Haut vor dem Anlegen des Tapes entfetten. Hierzu eignen sich Alkohol, Wundbenzin oder kalter schwarzer Kaffee.

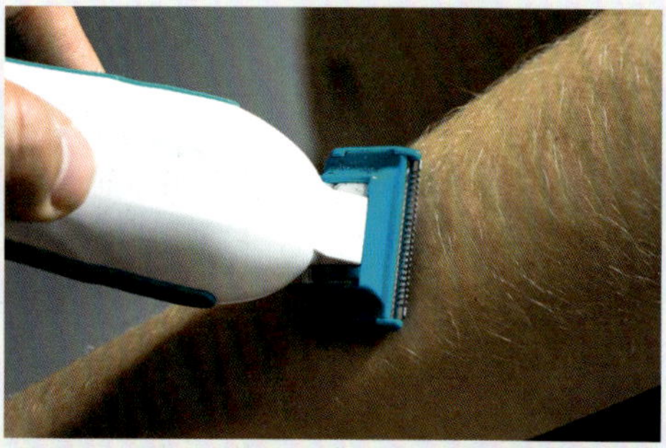

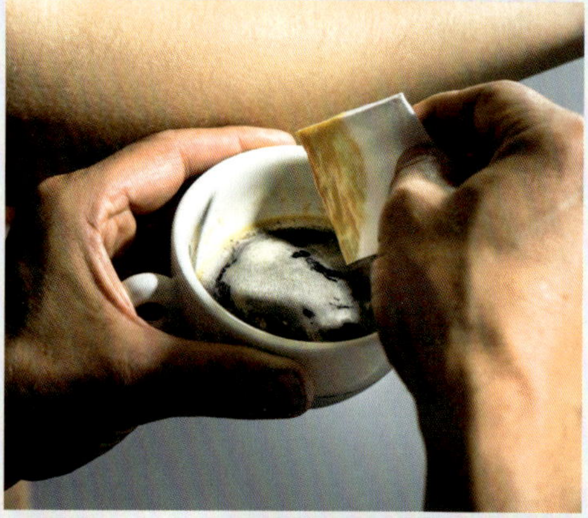

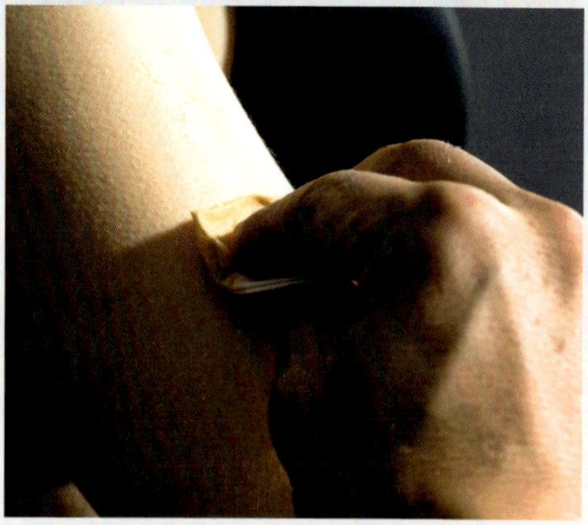

Warum Kaffee?

Ein sauberes Tuch in kalten schwarzen Kaffee tauchen, anschließend das gewünschte Hautareal mit dem getränkten Tuch abreiben und antrocknen lassen. Der Kaffee verbleibt auf der Haut. Jetzt kann getapt werden!

Ist die Haut nach mehrmaligem Tapen gereizt, sorgt der Kaffee ebenfalls für eine schnelle Erholung des betroffenen Hautareals.

Tipp: Hilft auch sehr gut bei Sonnenbrand oder wunder Haut (Babypopo)!

Before application

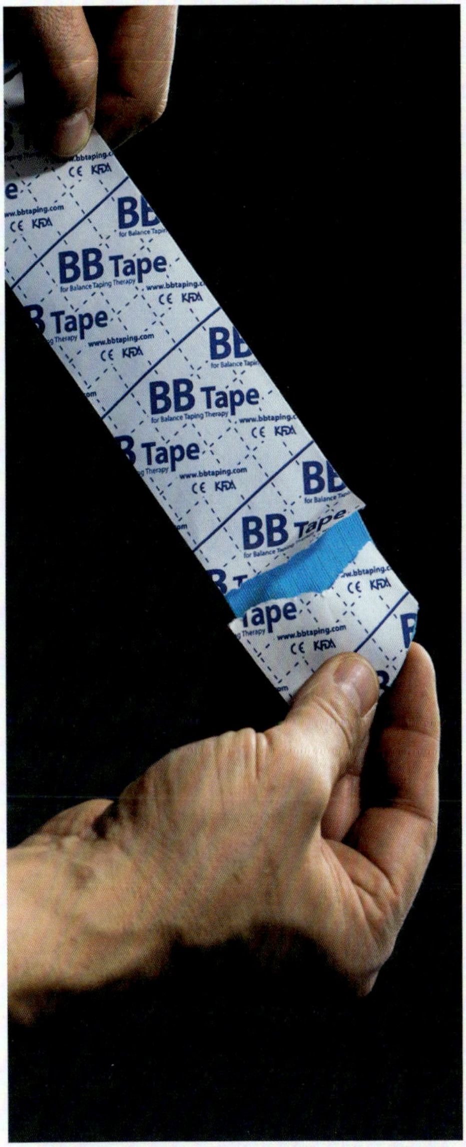

Please note the following before applying the tape strips:

- The skin must be dry.
- Hair should either be trimmed or shaved off.
- Remove any oil and grease from the skin before attaching. Alcohol, surgical spirit or cold coffee are all suitable for this.

Why coffee?

Dip a clean cloth in cold black coffee, then rub the desired area of skin with the saturated cloth and allow to dry. The coffee is left on the skin. Taping can now take place.

If the skin becomes irritated after being taped repeatedly, the coffee will also help the area concerned to recover rapidly.

Tip: Also very helpful for sunburn or sore skin (babies' bottoms)!

Das Aufbringen

Aufbringen in 6 Schritten

1 Das Trennpapier einreißen (siehe Foto) und das Papier auf den ersten 5 cm vom Tape ablösen.

2 Tape ohne Zug auflegen.

3 Trennpapier bis auf die letzten 5 cm entfernen.

4 Tape entweder mit oder ohne Zug (nur bei Ligamenttechniken) auf die vorgedehnte Muskulatur aufkleben.

5 Zum Schluss das letzte Stück Trennpapier entfernen und das Ende (Basis) aufkleben.

6 Das gesamte Tape sehr gut anreiben.

Hinweise

- Das Tape nach dem Aufkleben gut anreiben oder mit einem Fön erwärmen. Der Kleber benötigt Wärme, um sich optimal mit der Hautoberfläche verbinden zu können.

- In den ersten 2 Stunden nach der Applikation sollte der Patient vorsichtig mit den Tapekanten umgehen (Tape könnte sich lösen).

- Nach 2 Stunden kann das Tape voll belastet werden und mit Wasser in Kontakt kommen.

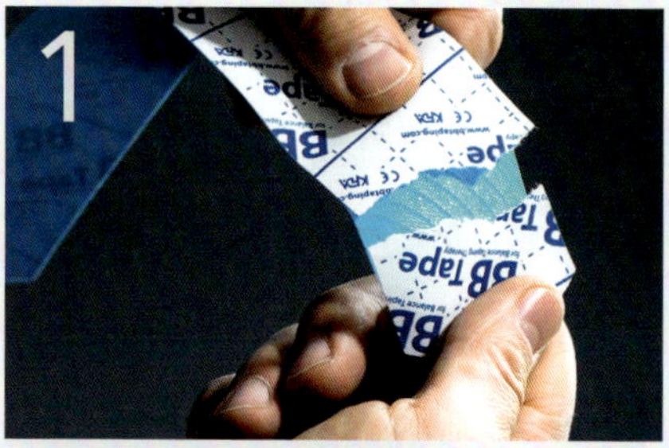

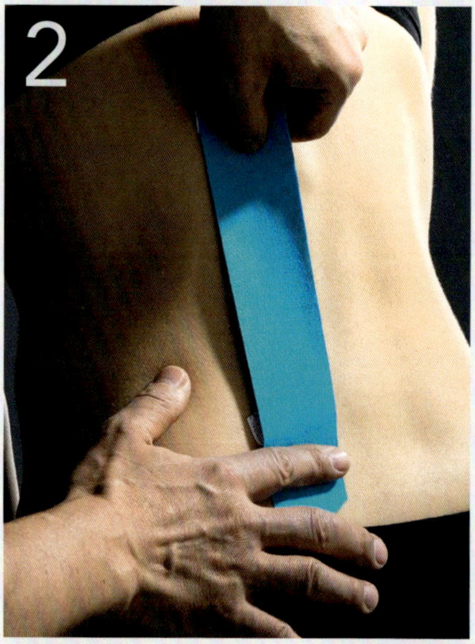

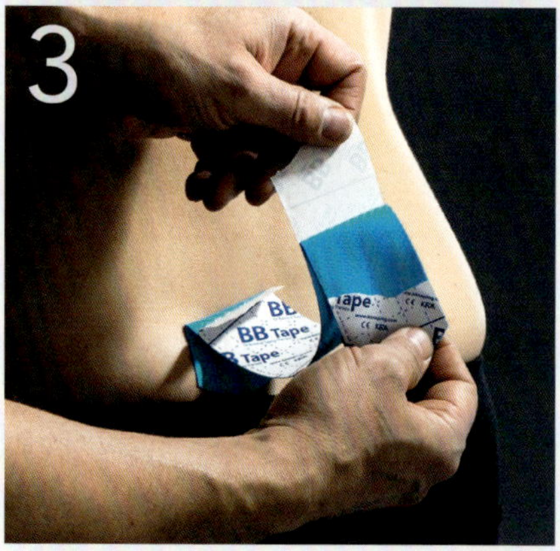

Application

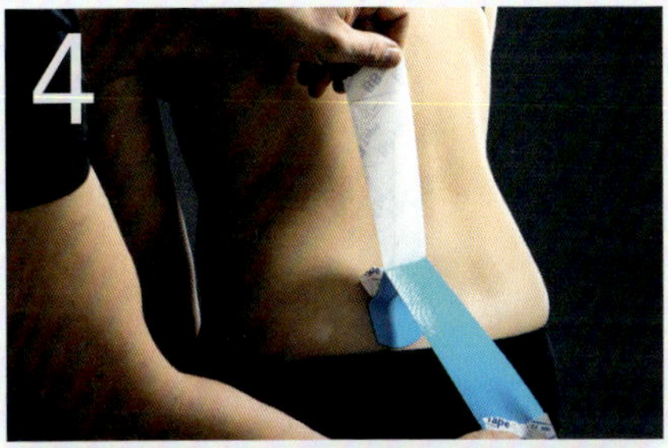

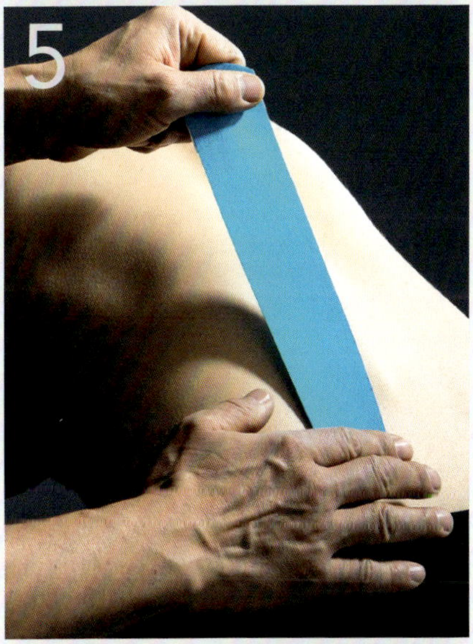

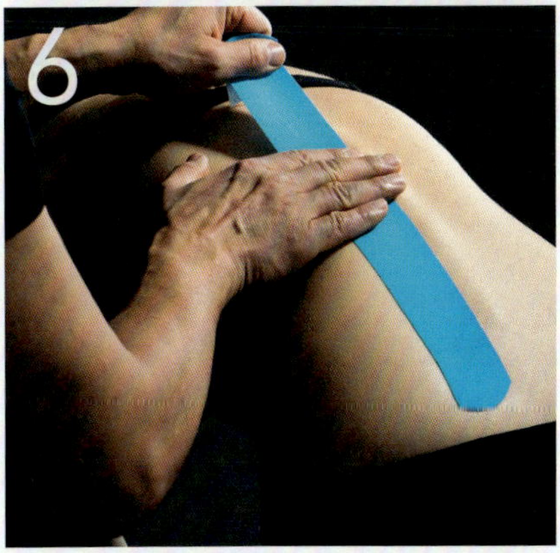

Apply in 6 stages

1 Tear the backing paper (see photo) and peel the first 5 cm of the paper away from the tape.

2 Apply the tape without stretch.

3 Remove the backing paper as far as the last 5 cm.

4 Affix the tape to the pre-stretched muscle either with stretch or without (ligament techniques only).

5 Finally, remove the last piece of backing paper and affix the end (base).

6 Rub down the whole of the tape very well.

Advice

- After affixing the tape, rub it down very well or warm it with a hair dryer. The adhesive needs warmth to bond optimally to the skin's surface.

- The patient should treat the edges of the tape with care for the first 2 hours after application (the tape could become loose).

- After 2 hours, the tape can be fully loaded and contacted with water.

Wasser und das Ablösen des Tapes

Wasser ist kein Problem

Auch Duschen, Schwimmen und Schwitzen ist für getapte Patienten möglich.

- Die klebenden Tapebänder sollten jedoch immer gut ausgespült werden, um Hautreaktionen und -irritationen zu vermeiden.
- Nach spätestens 7 Tagen sollte das Tape aus hygienischen Gründen gewechselt werden.

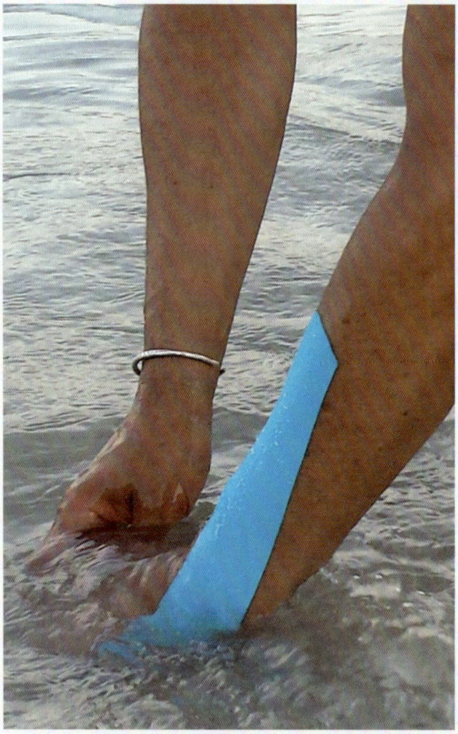

Tape schmerzfrei ablösen

Tapebänder mit etwas Öl oder Händedesinfektionslösung tränken und ca. 1–2 Minuten einziehen lassen. Anschließend kann das Tape mit leichtem Zug einfach entfernt werden.

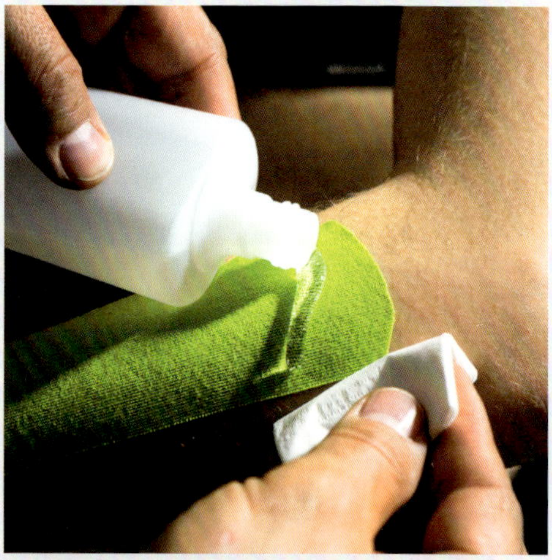

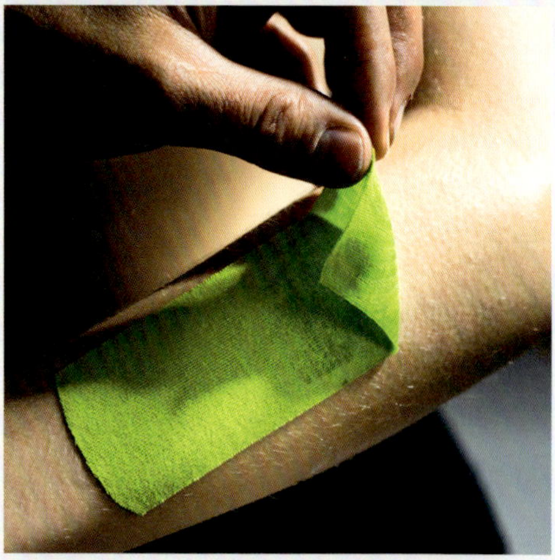

Water and removing the tape

Water is not a problem

Taped patients may also shower, swim and sweat.

- However, the adhesive tape strips should always be washed off well to prevent skin reactions and irritation.
- For hygiene reasons, the tape should be replaced after 7 days at the latest.

Painless tape removal

Saturate the tape strips with a little oil or hand disinfectant and leave to soak in for about 1-2 minutes. The tape can then be easily removed by tugging on it gently.

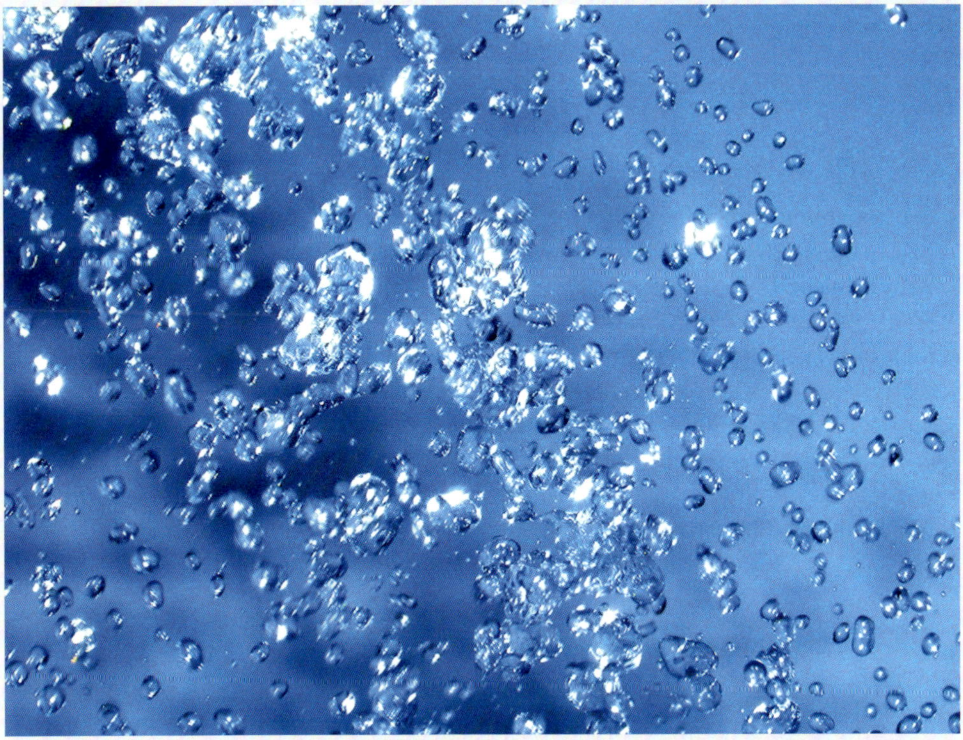

Überreaktionen

Nur so viele Tapebänder wie notwendig anlegen. (Weniger ist mehr!)

Zu viele Tapes können zu reflektorischen Überreaktionen des Organismus führen.

Typische Symptome

- Unwohlsein
- Schüttelfrost
- Gliederschmerzen
- Kopfschmerzen

Kontra-indikationen

- Schwangere nicht um den Bauchnabel herum tapen. Zu viele Reize könnten das Baby erreichen
- Kein Tape auf erkrankter Haut
- Vorsicht bei Pergamenthaut (Kortison)
- Vorsicht bei Patienten, die zu Hämatomen neigen (Blutverdünner)

Hyperreactions

Apply only as many tape strips as necessary. (Less is more!)

Too many tapes can cause reflex hyperreactions by the body.

Typical symptoms

- Feeling unwell
- Chills
- Joint pain
- Headaches

Contra-indications

- Do not tape pregnant women around the navel. Too many stimuli could reach the baby
- Do not tape diseased skin
- Take care on parchment skin (cortisone)
- Take care with patients who are prone to bruising (blood thinners)

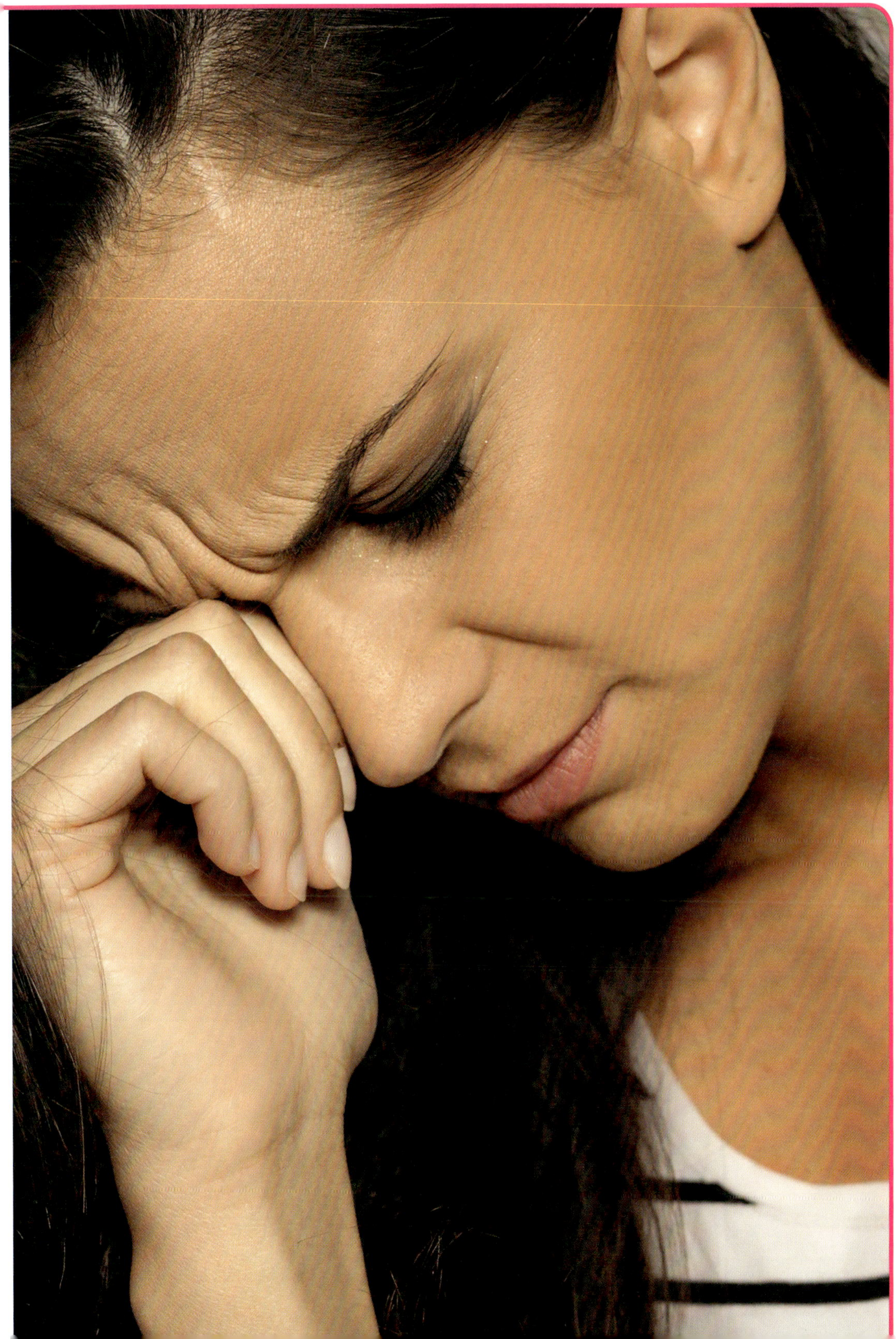

Die Schnitttechniken
Cutting techniques

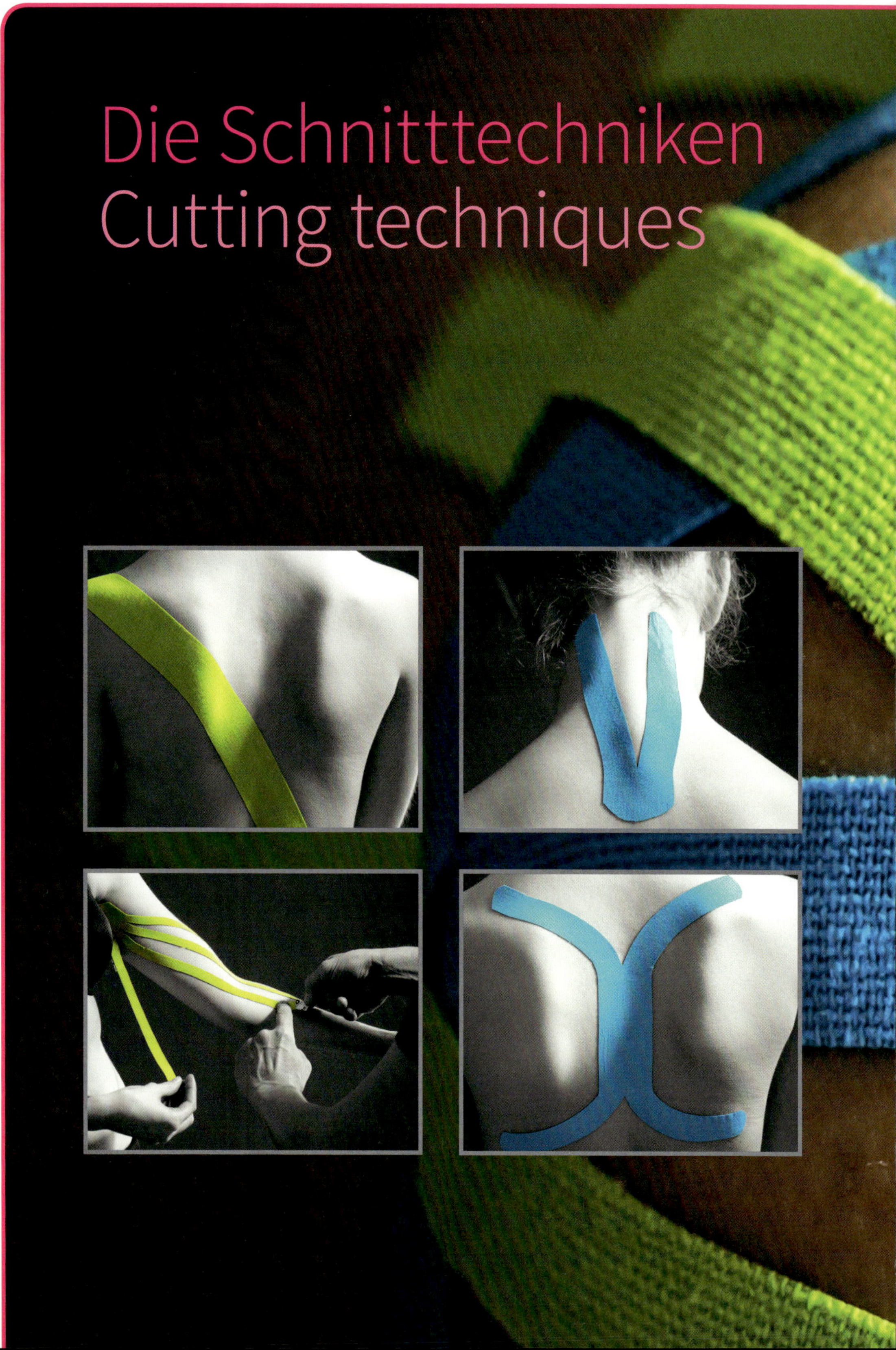

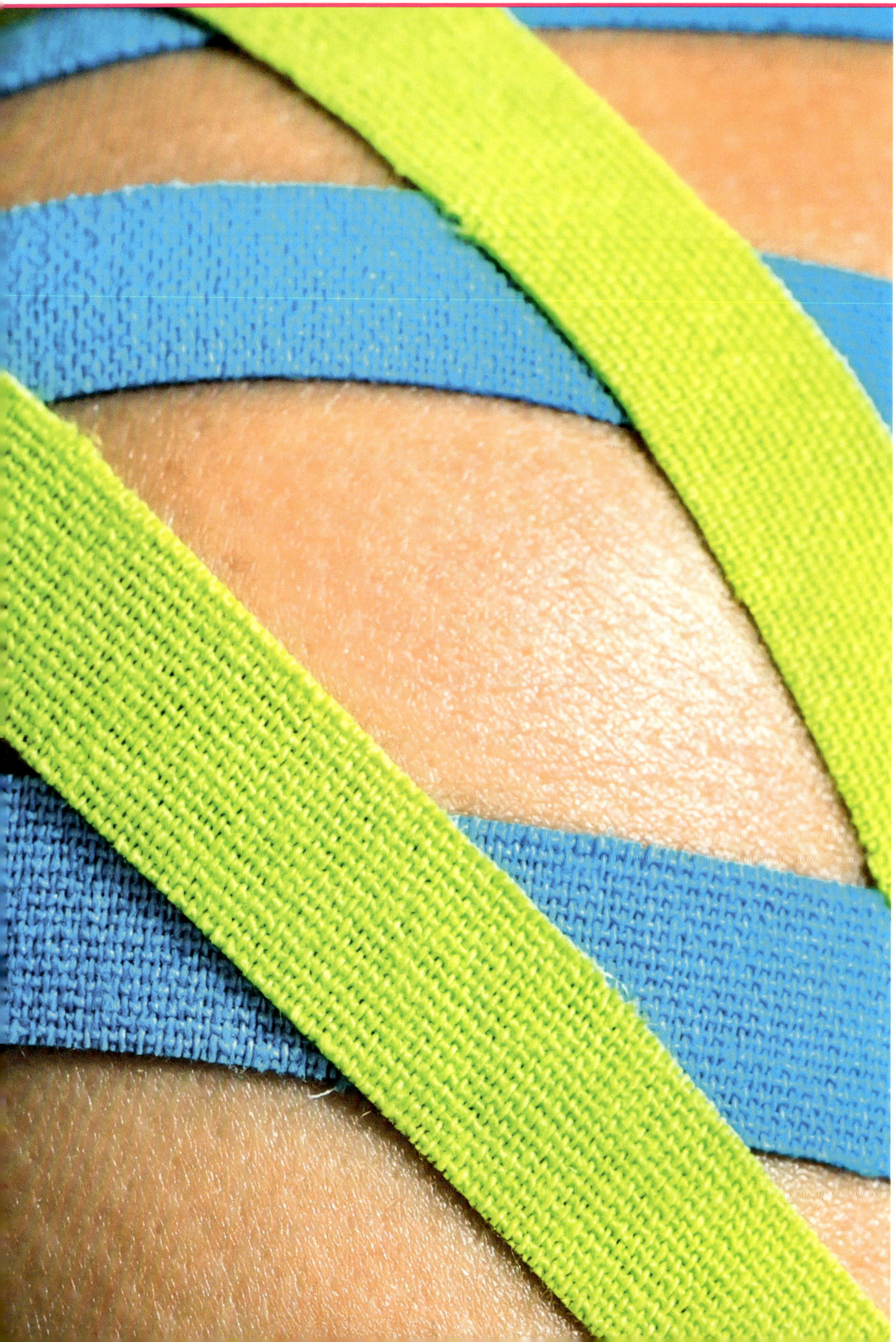

Kompakt-Technik

Tape wird nicht eingeschnitten

Anwendungsgebiete

- Muskelversorgung
- Korrekturtechniken

Compact technique

The tape is not cut

Indications

- Treatment of muscles
- Corrective techniques

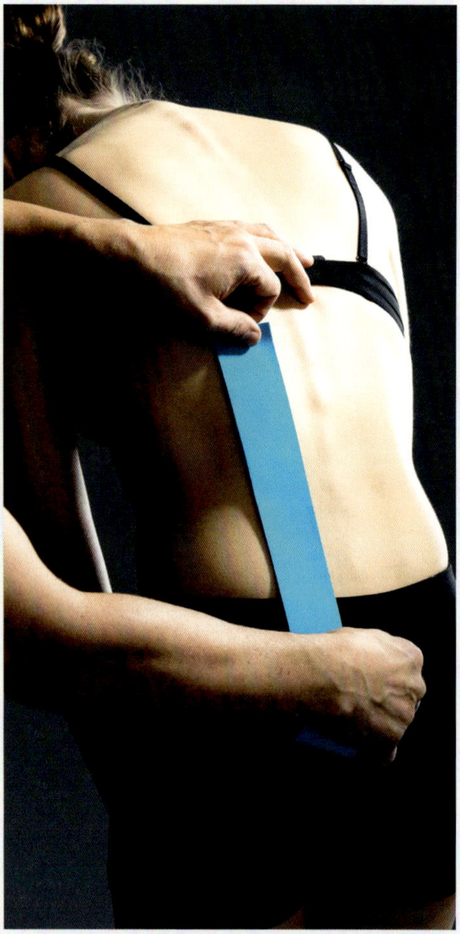

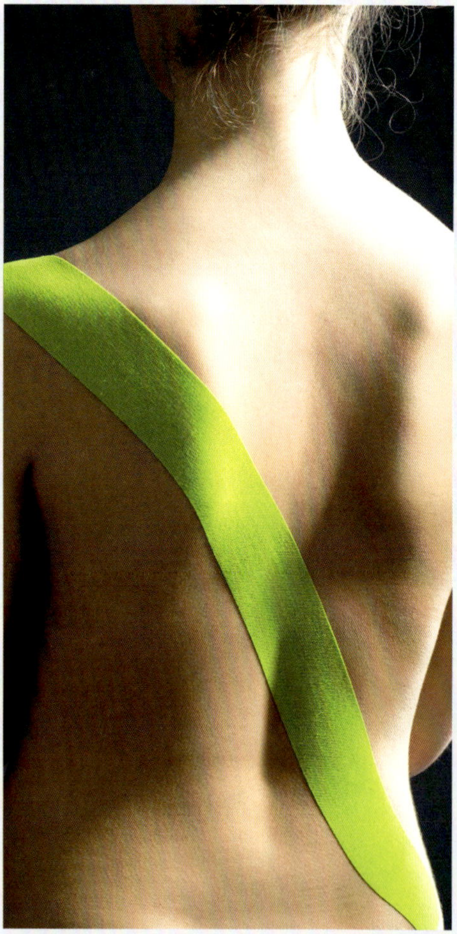

Y-Technik

Y-strip technique

Tape wird von einer Seite eingeschnitten

The tape is not cut

Anwendungsgebiete

- Muskelversorgungen
  Wird ein Areal umklebt, befindet sich die Wirkung des Tapes zusätzlich auch zwischen den Tapezügeln. Somit lassen sich Muskelbäuche umkleben, um den Muskel zu beeinflussen oder Wirkungen unter der Patella sowie unter dem Schulterblatt erzielen.
- Faszienversorgungen
- Entlastungstechniken

Indications

- Treatment of muscles
  If tape is affixed around an area, the tape also affects the areas between the tape tails. Therefore, tape can be affixed around muscle bellies to influence the muscle or to achieve effects underneath the patella and underneath the shoulder blade.
- Treatment of the fascia
- Decompression techniques

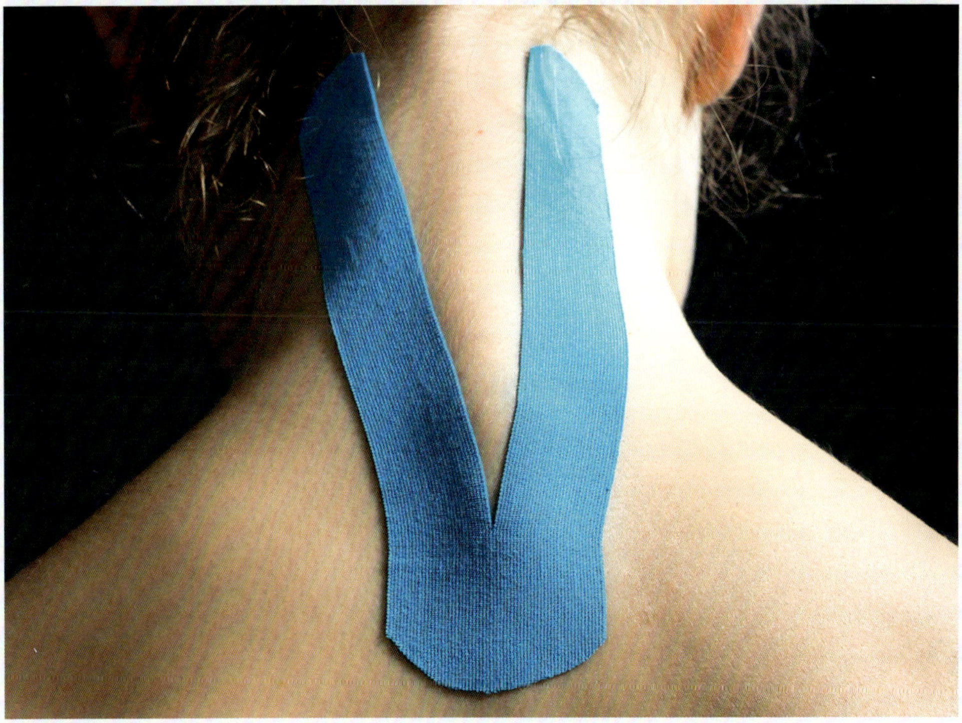

Fächer-Technik

Tape wird mehrmals eingeschnitten

Durch das mehrfache Einschneiden lässt sich ein größeres Hautareal abdecken. Dünne Tapestreifen haben nur noch einen Effekt auf das Lymphgefäßsystem, nicht mehr auf die Muskulatur.

Anwendungsgebiete

- Klassische Lymphtechnik

Fan-cut technique

The tape is cut several times

Cutting the tape several times means that a larger area of skin can be covered. It has also been noticed that thin tape strips have an effect only on the lymphatic system and that the muscles do not respond to the tape.

Indications

- Classic lymphatic technique

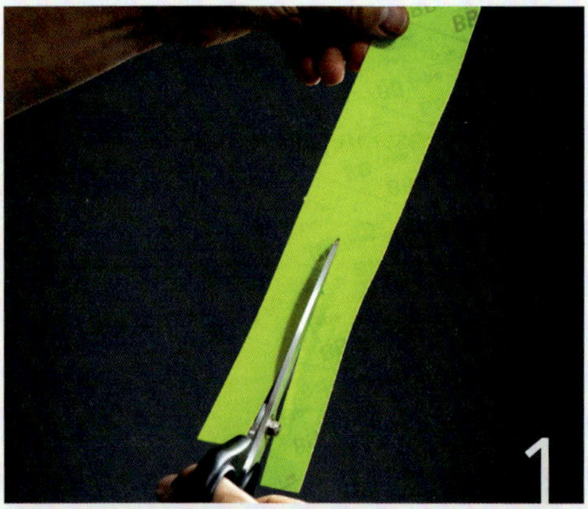

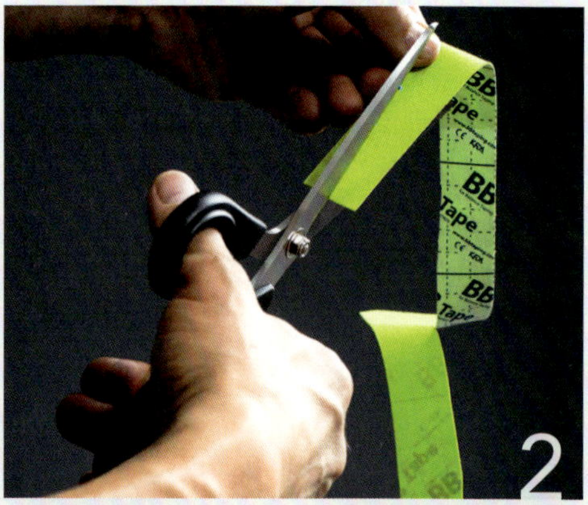

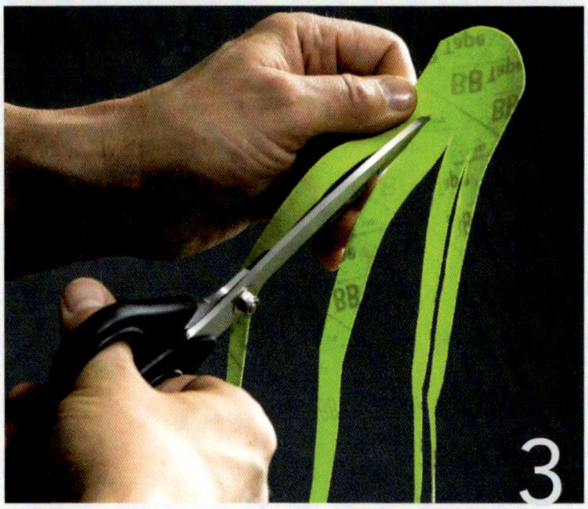

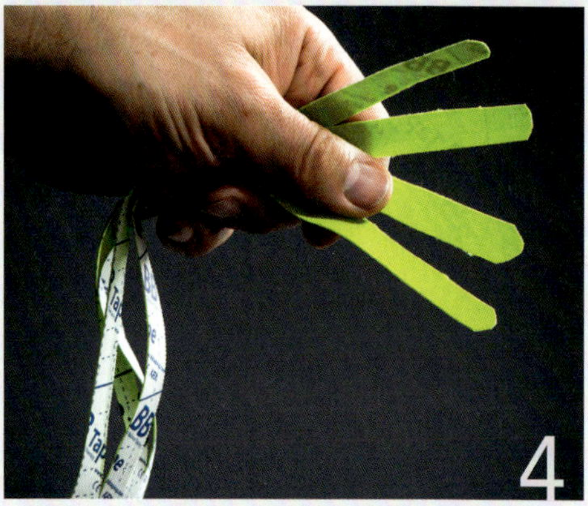

Enden abrunden

Round off the ends

X-Technik

Tape wird von beiden Seiten eingeschnitten

Selten benutzte Technik.

Anwendungsgebiete

- Areale mit wenig Fläche zum Kleben
- besondere Versorgungstechniken z. B. auf Reflexzonen

X-tape technique

The tape is cut from both sides

A rarely used technique.

Indications

- Areas with little space to affix tape or
- Special treatment techniques, e.g. on reflex zones

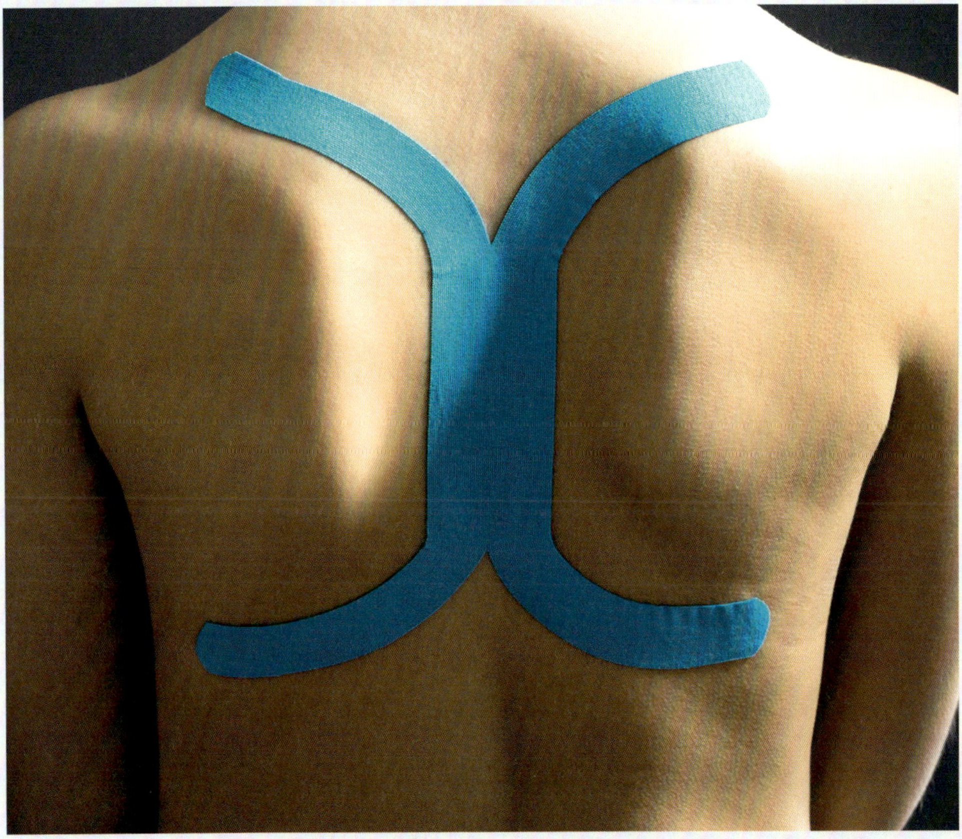

Die Klebetechniken
Taping techniques

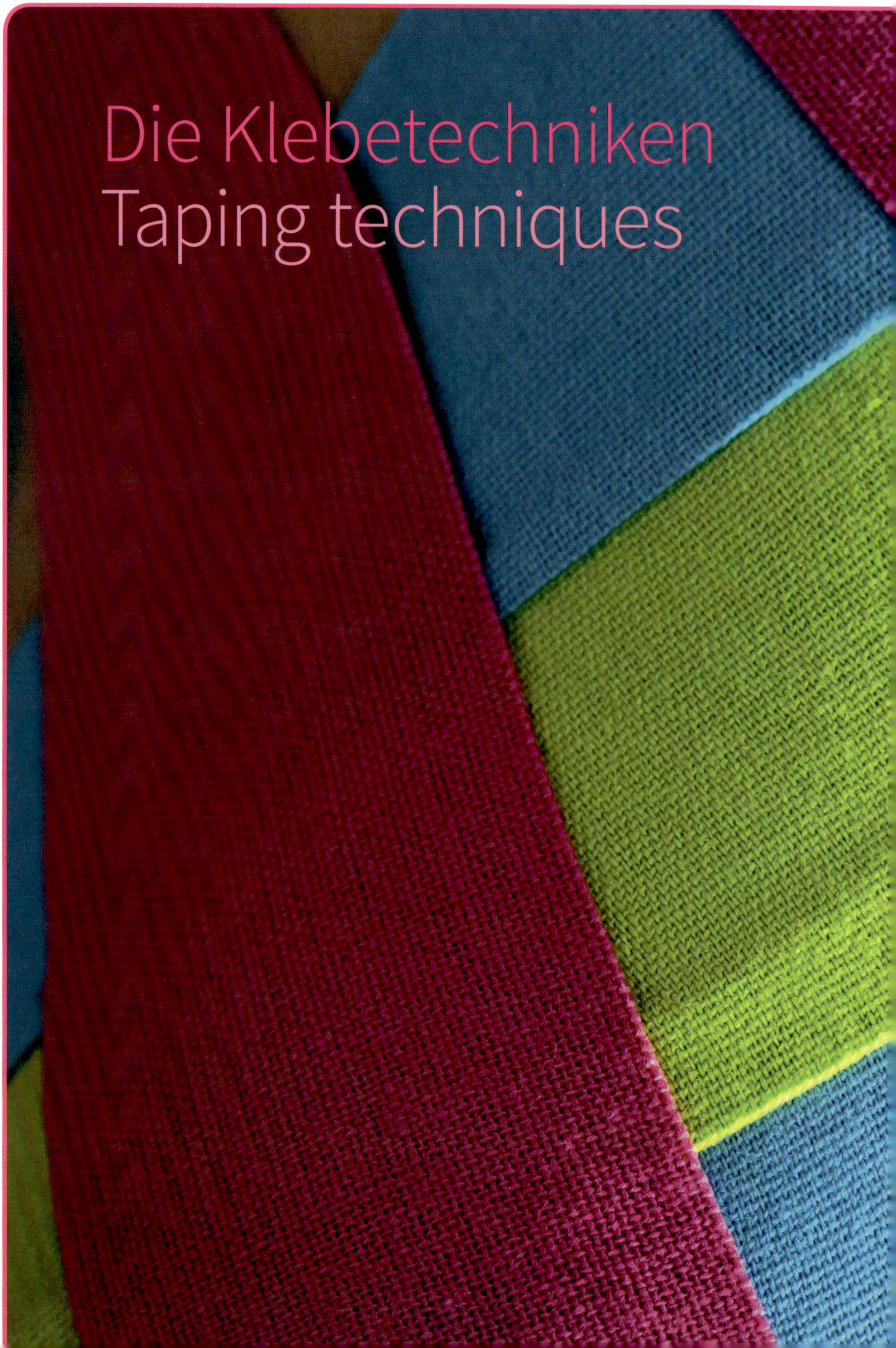

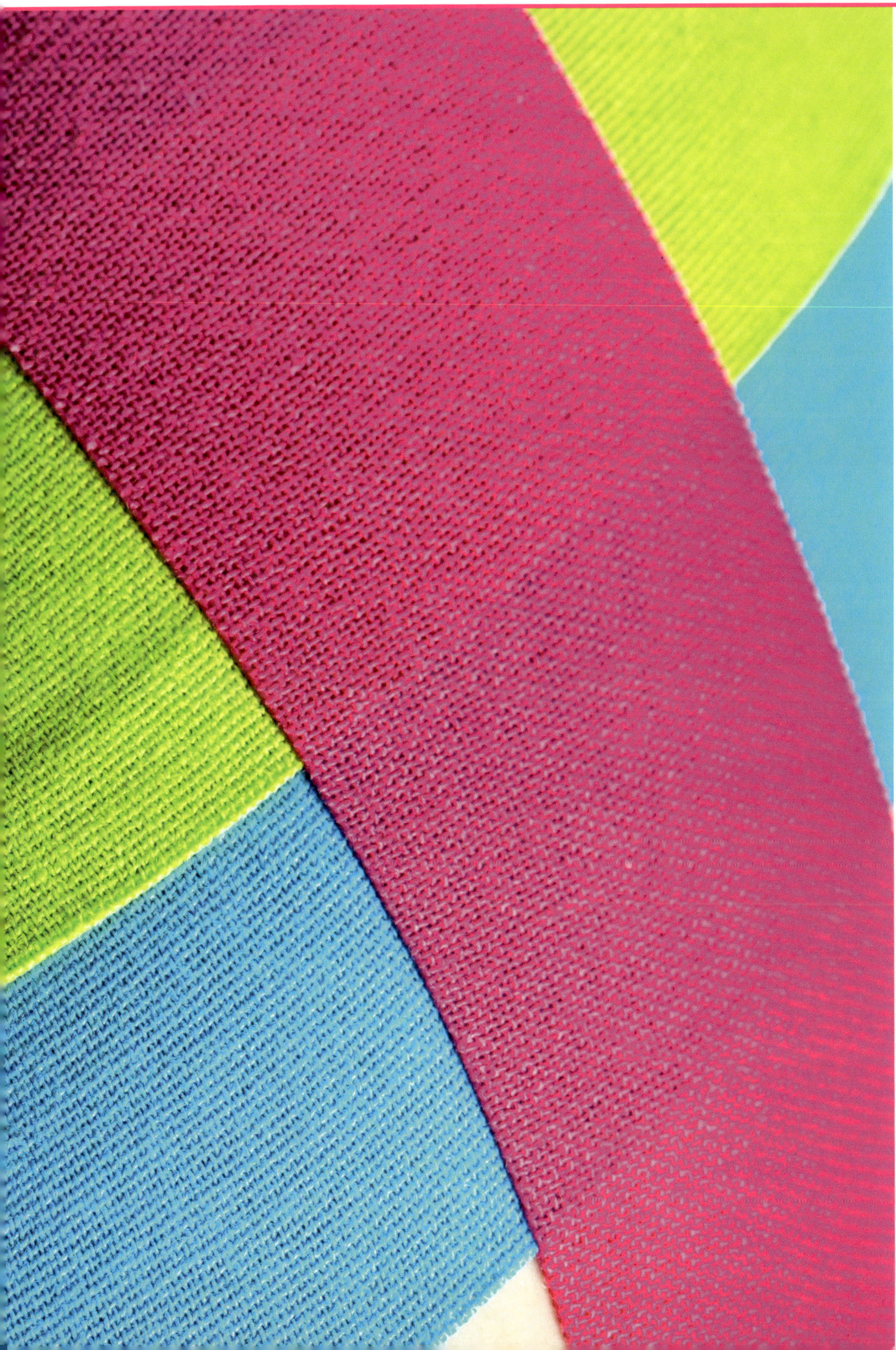

Muskeltechnik
Muscle technique

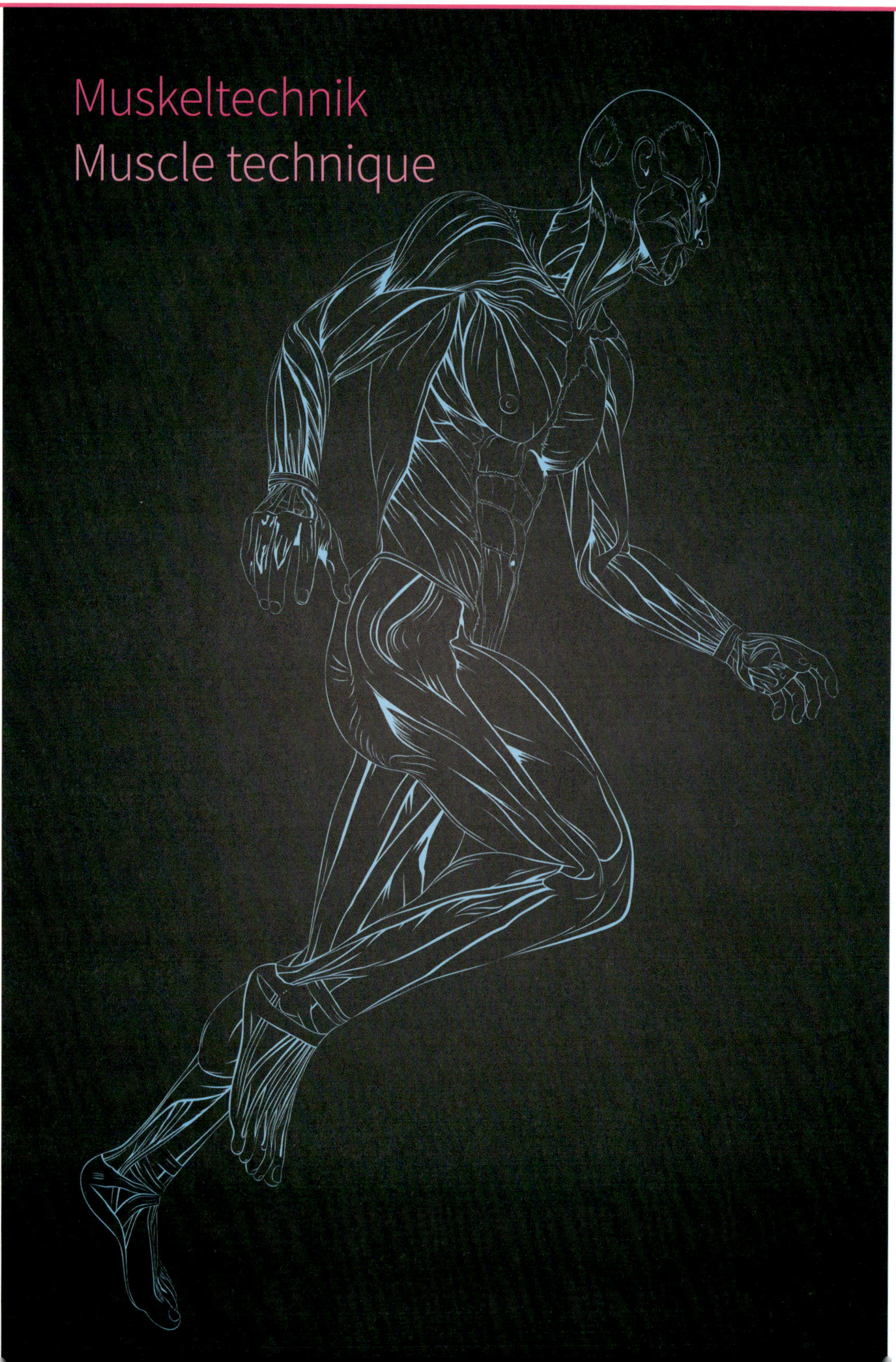

Wirkungen

Der Muskel kann in der Dehnung oder Kontraktion unterstützt werden.

Bitte beachten:

Bei allen Schmerzzuständen, Muskelverspannungen etc. muss der Muskel entlastend, **detonisierend**, getapt werden.

Bei allen Versorgungen, bei denen z. B. ein Gelenk stabilisiert oder die Muskelkontraktion angeregt werden soll, muss der Muskel **tonisierend** getapt werden.

Effects

The muscle can be assisted with stretching or contracting.

Please note:

In the case of all painful conditions, muscle strains, etc., the muscle must be taped to achieve decompression, **decreased tone**.

In the case of all treatments where, for example, a joint has to be stabilised or muscle contraction stimulated, the muscle must be taped to achieve **increased tone**.

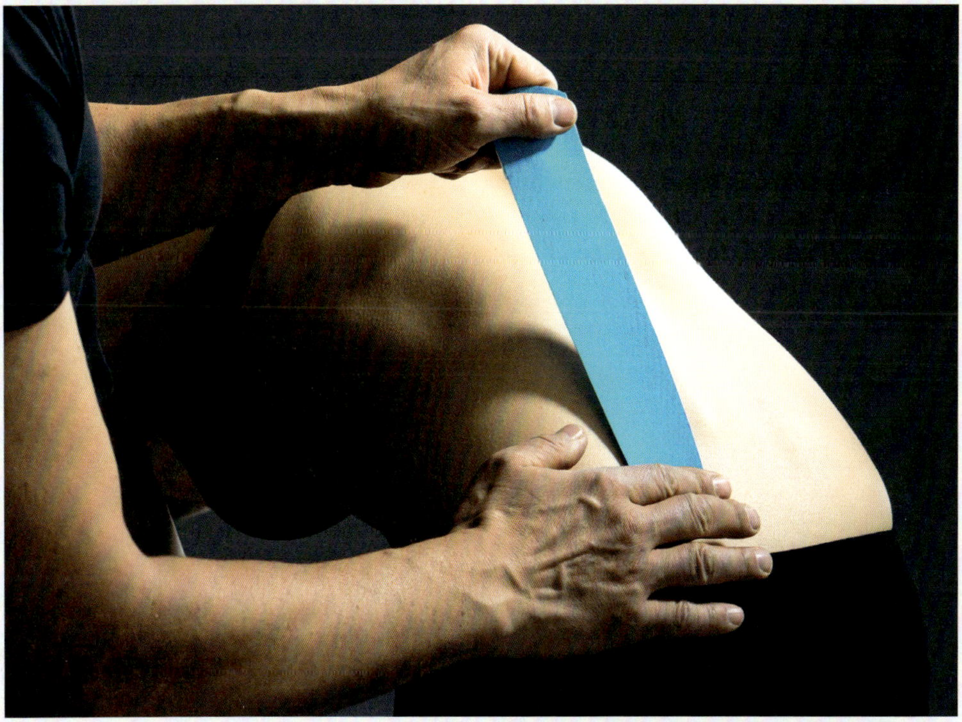

Detonisierende Wirkung

(unterstützt die Muskeldehnung und lindert Schmerzen auf gestörter Muskulatur)

Entlastungstechnik für den Muskel

Wirkungen

Wirkt schmerzentlastend, der Muskel kann weiter gedehnt werden (kann Verletzungen im Sport vorbeugen), kann zur besseren Mobilisation beitragen und erhöht den Stoffwechsel im Muskel.

Tape bitte immer am unteren oder äußeren Ende des Muskels starten.

Begründung

Das elastische Tape hat die Eigenschaft, sich nach dem Aufkleben immer wieder zur Basis (Startpunkt des Tapes) zurückziehen zu wollen. Diese Kleberichtung hat einen großen Einfluss auf das Schmerzempfinden des Patienten.

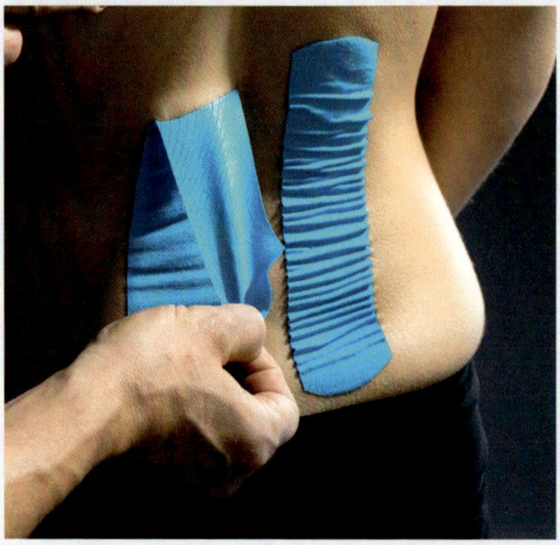

Anwendungsgebiete

Die detonisierende Technik wirkt schmerzlindernd und sollte bei allen Schmerzpatienten angewendet werden.

Beim Sport kann der Muskel auf Maximalkraft länger belastet werden. Der Muskel ermüdet nicht so schnell.

Technik

- Haut und Muskel vordehnen
- Tape ohne Zug auf die Haut aufkleben

Test

Sobald das Tape aufgeklebt ist und der vorgedehnte Muskel entlastet wird, muss das Tape die Haut sichtbar in Wellenform anheben.

Sind diese Wellen nicht zu sehen, wurde das Tape mit zu viel Zug aufgeklebt und die reflektorischen Reize des Tapes können nicht wirken.

Tone-decreasing effect

(assists muscle stretching and alleviate pain on defected muscles)

Decompression technique for muscles

Effects

Pain-relieving, the muscle is able to be stretched further (may prevent sports injuries), may contribute to better mobilisation.

Please always start the tape at the lower or outer edge of the muscle.

Reason

Elastic tape has the property of wanting to keep retracting to the base (tape starting point) once affixed. This direction of application has a great influence on the patient's perception of pain.

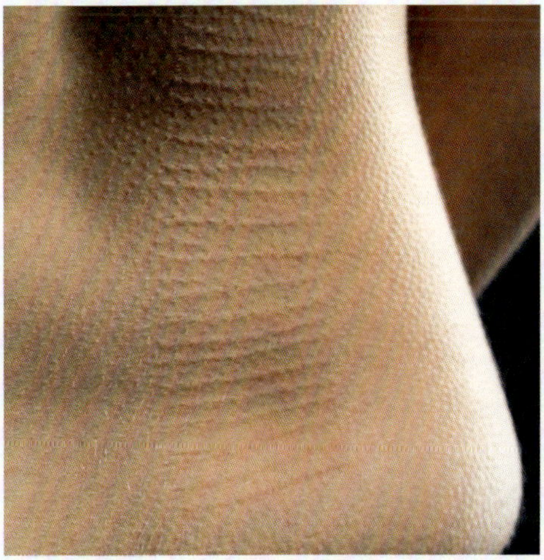

Indications

This technique is pain-relieving and should be applied to achieve decreased tone in all patients who are in pain.

During sport, the muscle can be loaded for longer at maximum force. The muscle does not become fatigued so rapidly.

Technique

- Pre-stretch the skin and muscle
- Affix the tape to the skin without stretch

Test

As soon as the tape is affixed and the pre-stretched muscle released, it must become visible that the tape lifts the skin in waves.

If these waves cannot be seen, the tape was affixed with too much stretch and the tape's reflex stimuli cannot act.

Tonisierende Wirkung (unterstützt die Muskelkontraktion)

Achtung: Darf nur bei Patienten mit wenig bis keinen Schmerzen aufgeklebt werden, da ansonsten das Schmerzempfinden stark zunehmen kann.

Wirkungen

Wirkt stabilisierend auf die Gelenke und kann korrigierend in den Bereichen Knie, Schulter, Rücken, Fuß und Sprunggelenk angewendet werden.

Anwendungsgebiete

- Haltungskorrektur am Rücken
- Schulterkorrektur (z. B. Paresen, Schulterinstabilität ...)
- Fußkorrektur (Knick-, Senk-, Spreizfuß)
- Kniestellungskorrektur (X- oder O-Bein)

Technik

- Muskelverkürzen (Ansatz und Ursprung annähern)
- Tape mit leichtem bis mittlerem Zug auf die Haut aufkleben

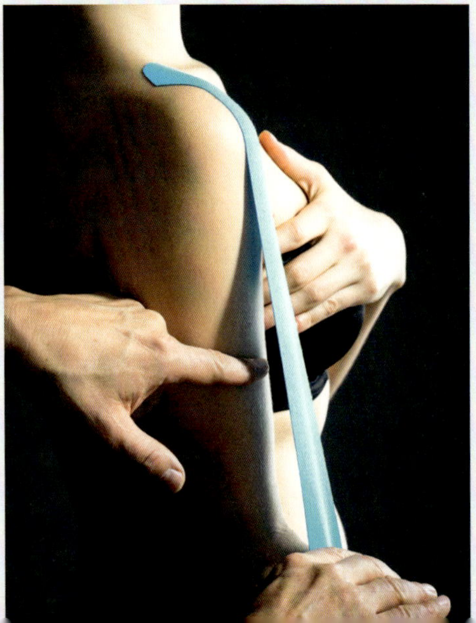

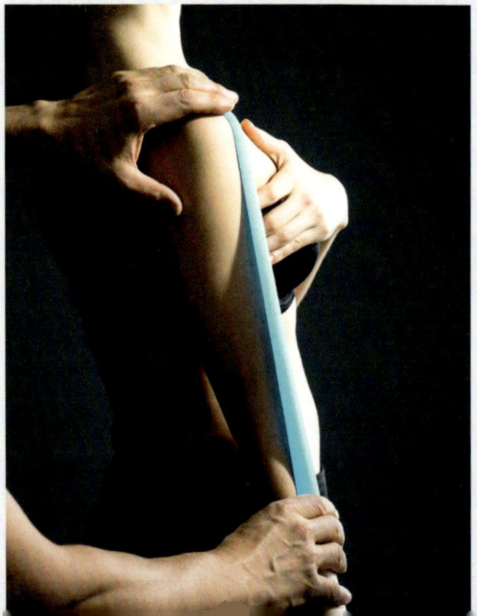

Tone-increasing effect (assists muscle contraction)

N.B.: Must be affixed only to patients with little or no pain, otherwise there may be a great increase in pain perception.

Effects

Has a stabilising effect on the joints and can be used correctively on the knee, shoulder, back, foot and ankle joint.

Indications

- Posture correction on the back
- Shoulder correction (e.g. palsy, shoulder instability, etc.)
- Foot correction (skewfoot, flat foot, splayfoot)
- Knee position correction (knock knees or bow legs)

Technique

- Shorten the muscle (bring the insertion and origin closer together)
- Affix the tape to the skin with slight to moderate stretch

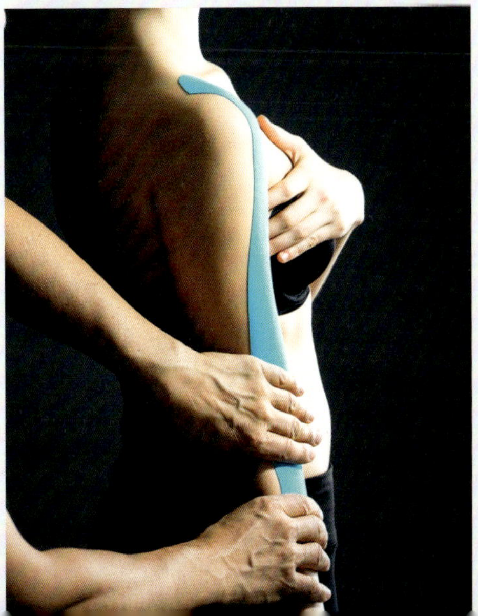

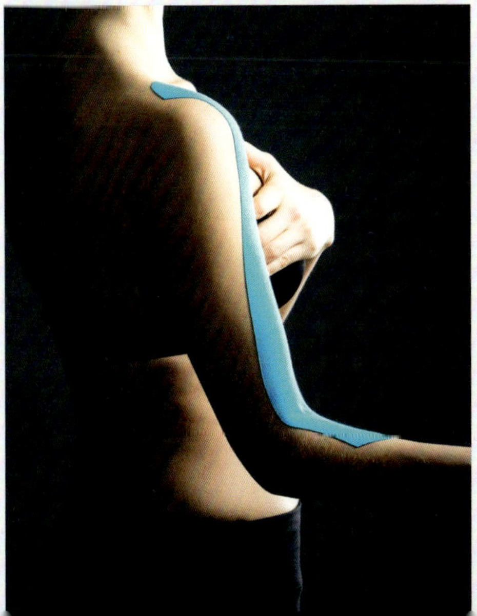

MUSKELTECHNIK – So wird‘s gemacht!
MUSCLE TECHNIQUE – That’s how it’s done!

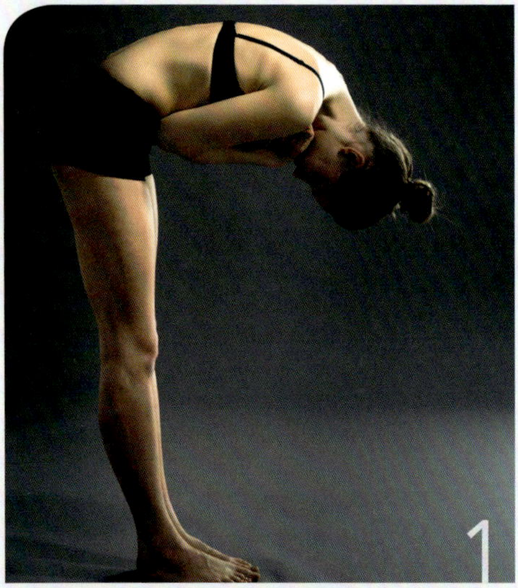

Haut des zu tapenden Areals so weit wie möglich dehnen

Stretch the skin on the area to be taped as far as possible

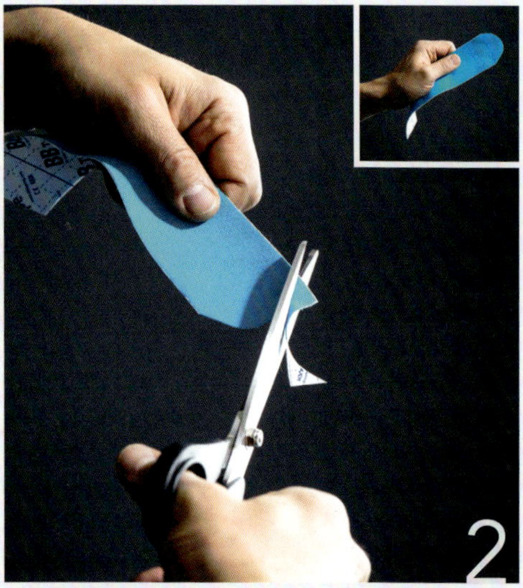

Tape an den Enden abrunden (damit es später länger hält)

Round off the ends of the tape (so that it stays in place longer later)

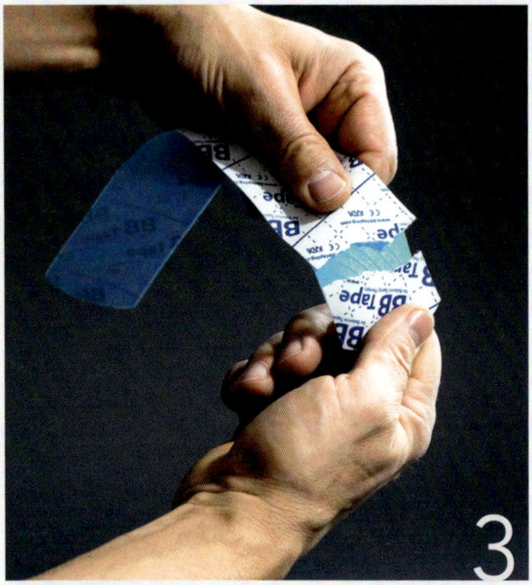

Tapetrennpapier nach ca. 5 cm quer einreißen (an beiden Enden des Tape)

Tear the tape backing paper crossways about 5 cm in (at both ends of the tape)

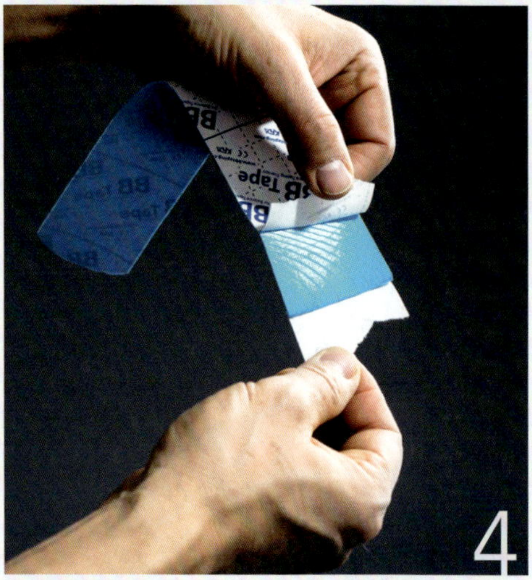

Papier an einem Ende entfernen

Remove the paper at one end

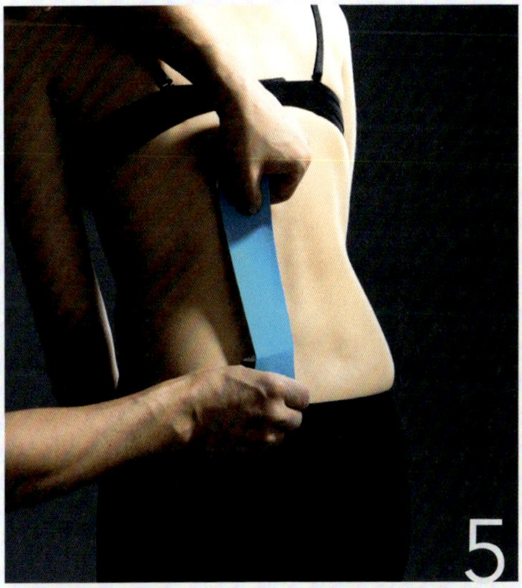

Tape mit dem vom Trennpapier befreiten Ende aufkleben

Affix the tape at the end from which the backing paper has been removed

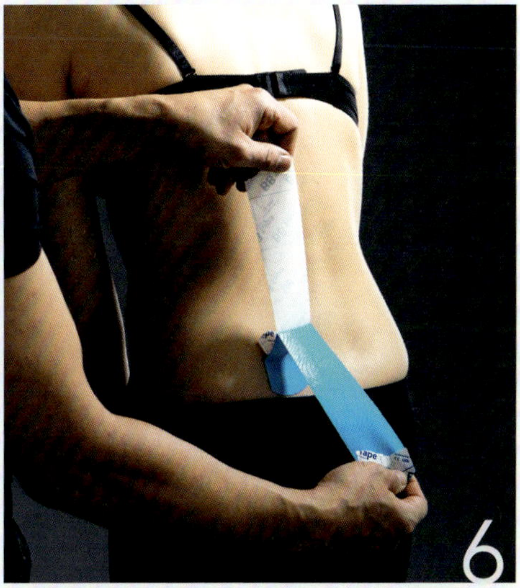

Mittleres Papier entfernen

Remove the middle section of the paper

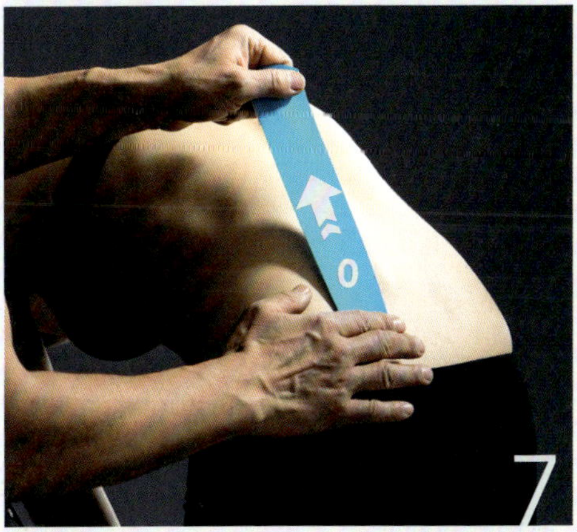

Tape, ohne daran zu ziehen, von unten nach oben auf die Haut anstreichen. Wichtig: Bitte nicht am Tape ziehen!

Smooth the tape on the skin in an upward direction without tugging on it Important: Please do not: tug on the tape!

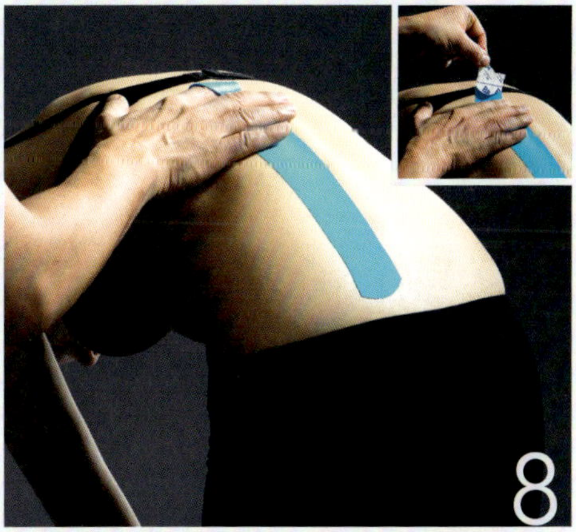

Befreien Sie das Ende des Tapes vom Papier und drücken es ohne Zug an. Gesamtes Tape auf der Haut anreiben bis eine leichte Wärme unter den Fingern zu spüren ist

Remove the end of the tape from the paper and press it down without tugging on it. Rub down all of the tape on the skin until slight warmth can be felt underneath the fingers

Ergebnis

Nach Entlastung der Muskeln muss das Tape die Haut in Wellen nach oben anheben können.

Nur dann können reflektorische Reize bewirkt und die Gefäße gedehnt werden.

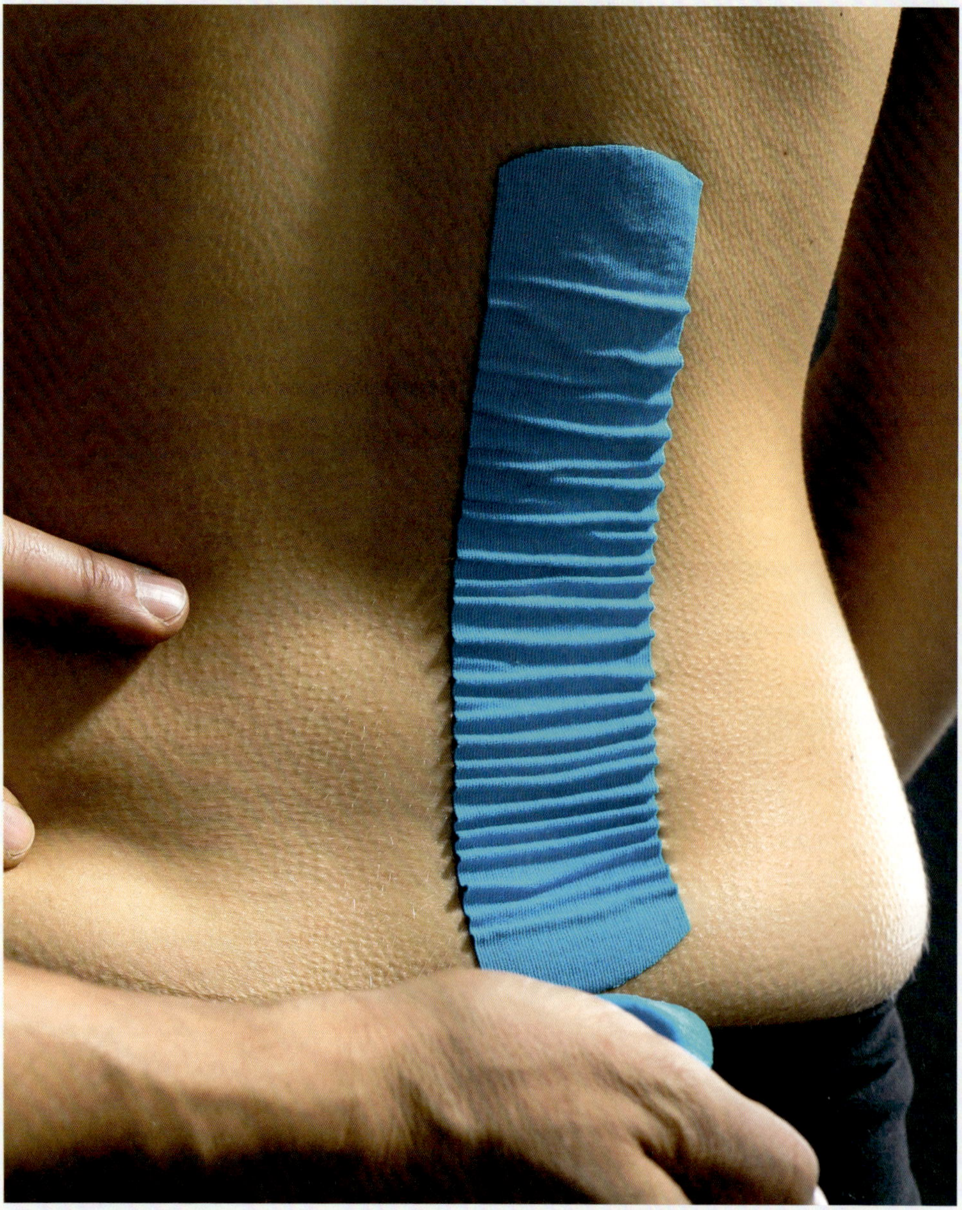

Result

Once the muscles relax, the tape must be able to lift the skin upwards in waves. Only in this way can reflex stimuli be produced and the vessels stretched.

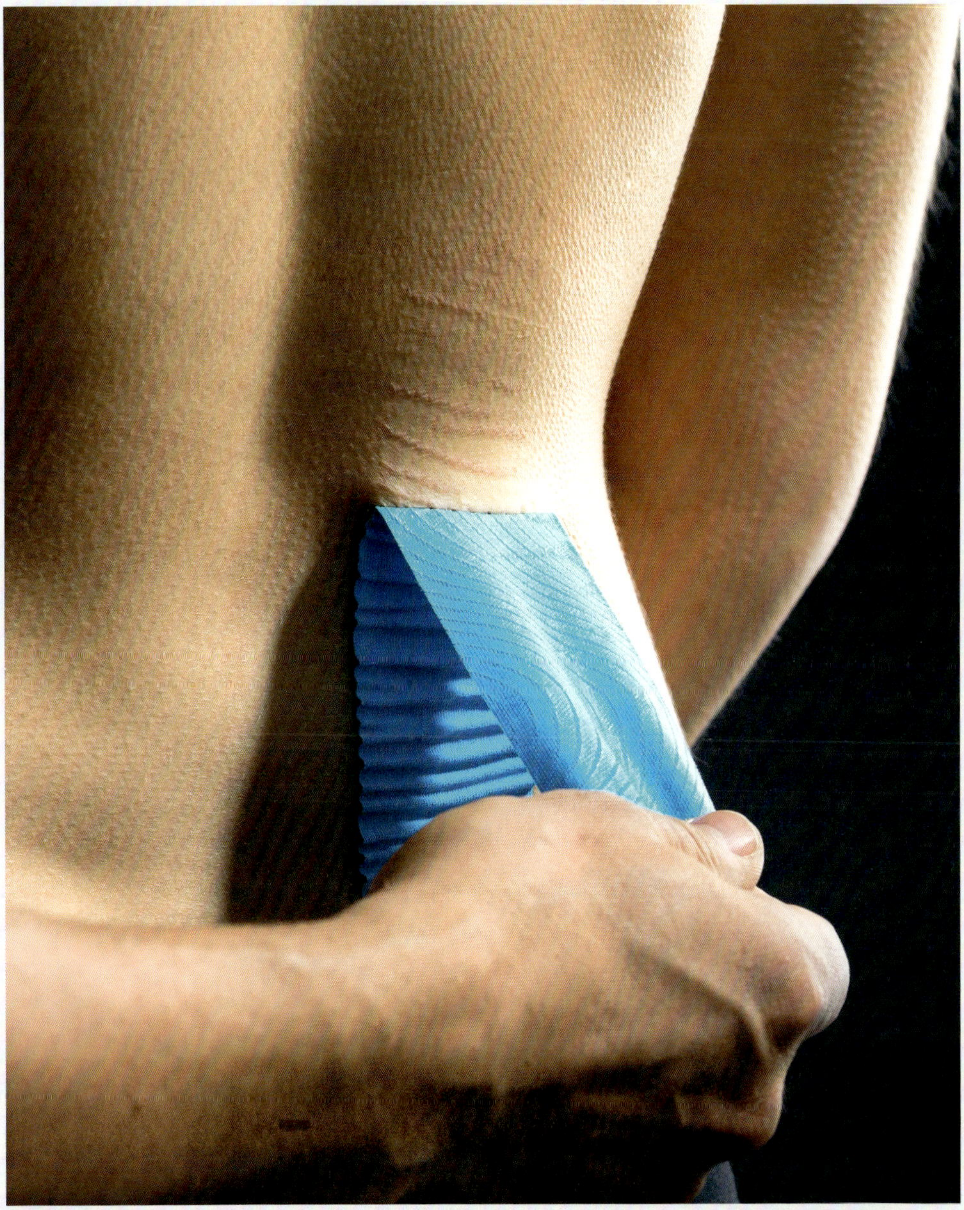

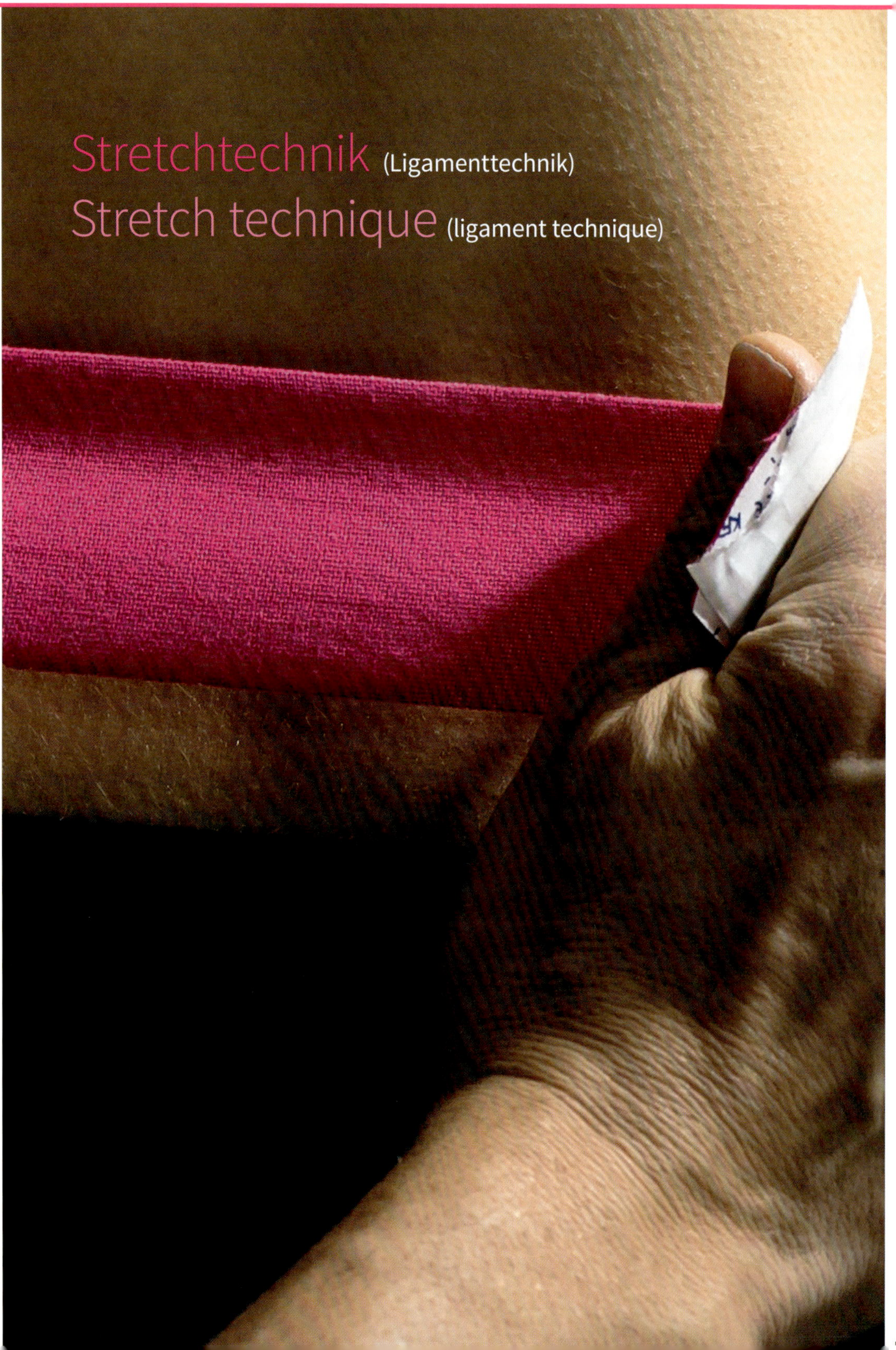
Stretchtechnik (Ligamenttechnik)
Stretch technique (ligament technique)

Wann wird diese Technik angewendet?

Diese Technik dient der Entlastung eines gesamten Areals.

Anwendungsgebiete

- Hämatome
- Schmerzpunkte
- Narben
- Gelenkspalt
- Entlastung der Patella
- Entlastung einzelner Wirbelkörper

When is this technique used?

This technique is used to decompress a whole area.

Indications

- Haematomas
- Painful spots
- Scars
- Joint space
- Patella decompression
- Decompression of individual vertebrae

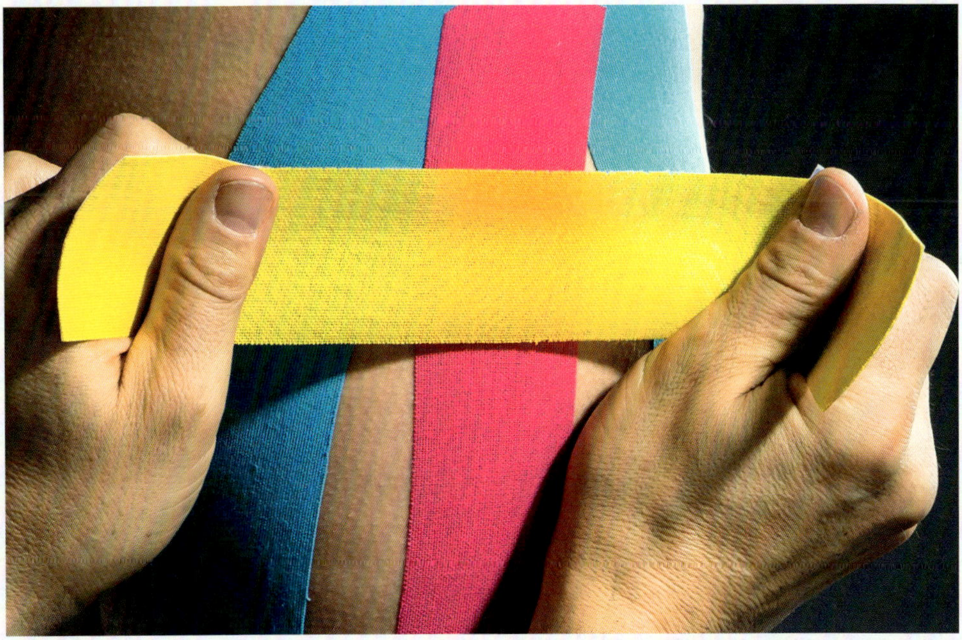

LIGAMENTTECHNIK – So wird's gemacht!
LIGAMENT TECHNIQUE – That's how it's done!

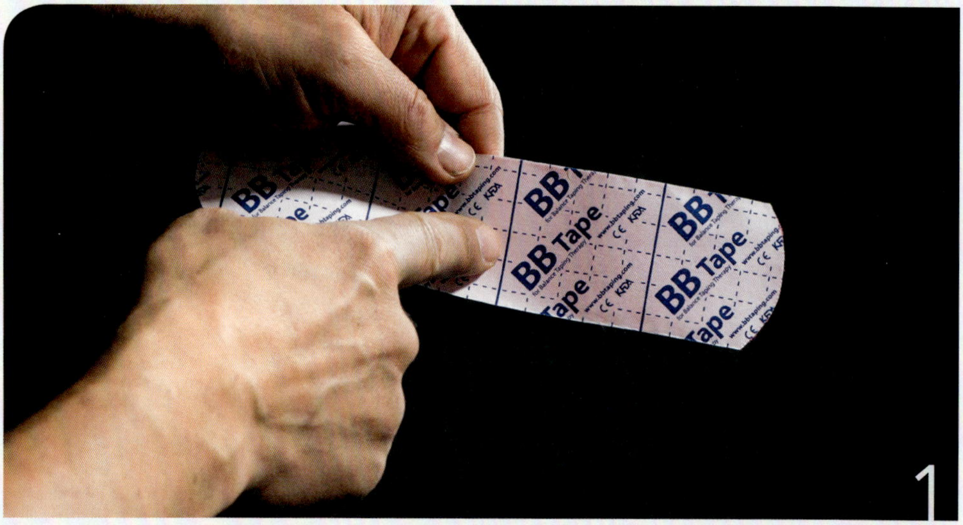

Papier in der Mitte des Tapezügels öffnen

Open the paper in the middle of the tape tail

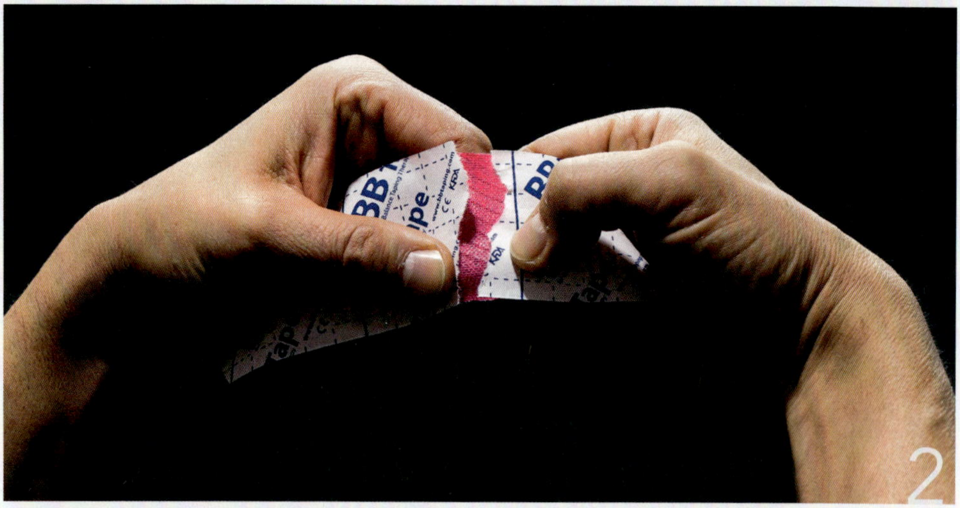

Tapetrennpapier von der Mitte aus zu beiden Seiten aufziehen

Lift the tape backing paper from the centre outwards on both sides

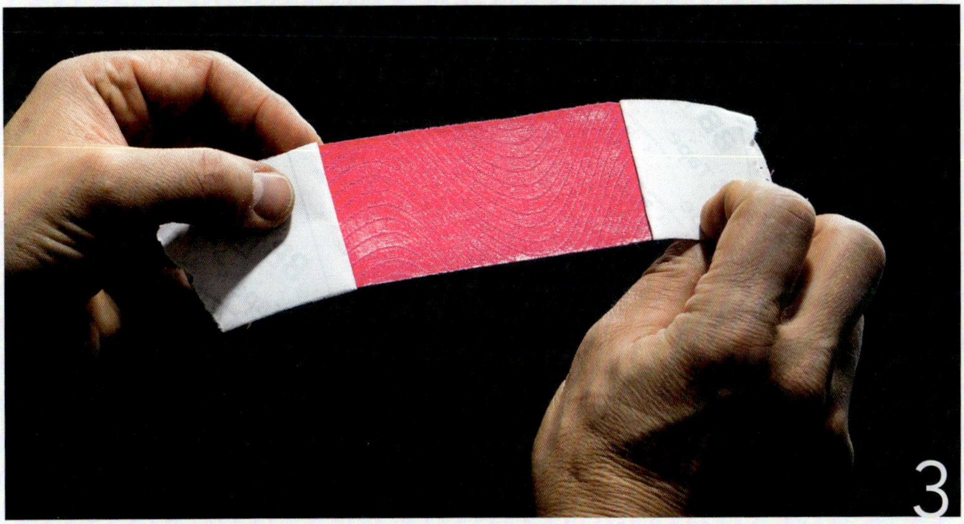

Tape kann je nach Areal und Indikation bis zu 100 % gedehnt werden

The tape can be stretched up to 100% depending on the area and indication

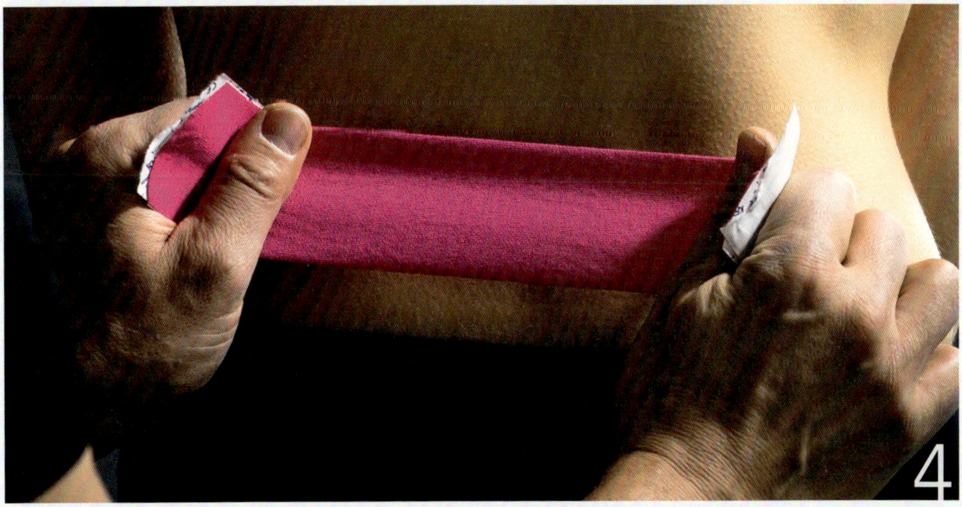

Tape aufkleben

Affix tape

Lymphtechnik
Lymphatic technique

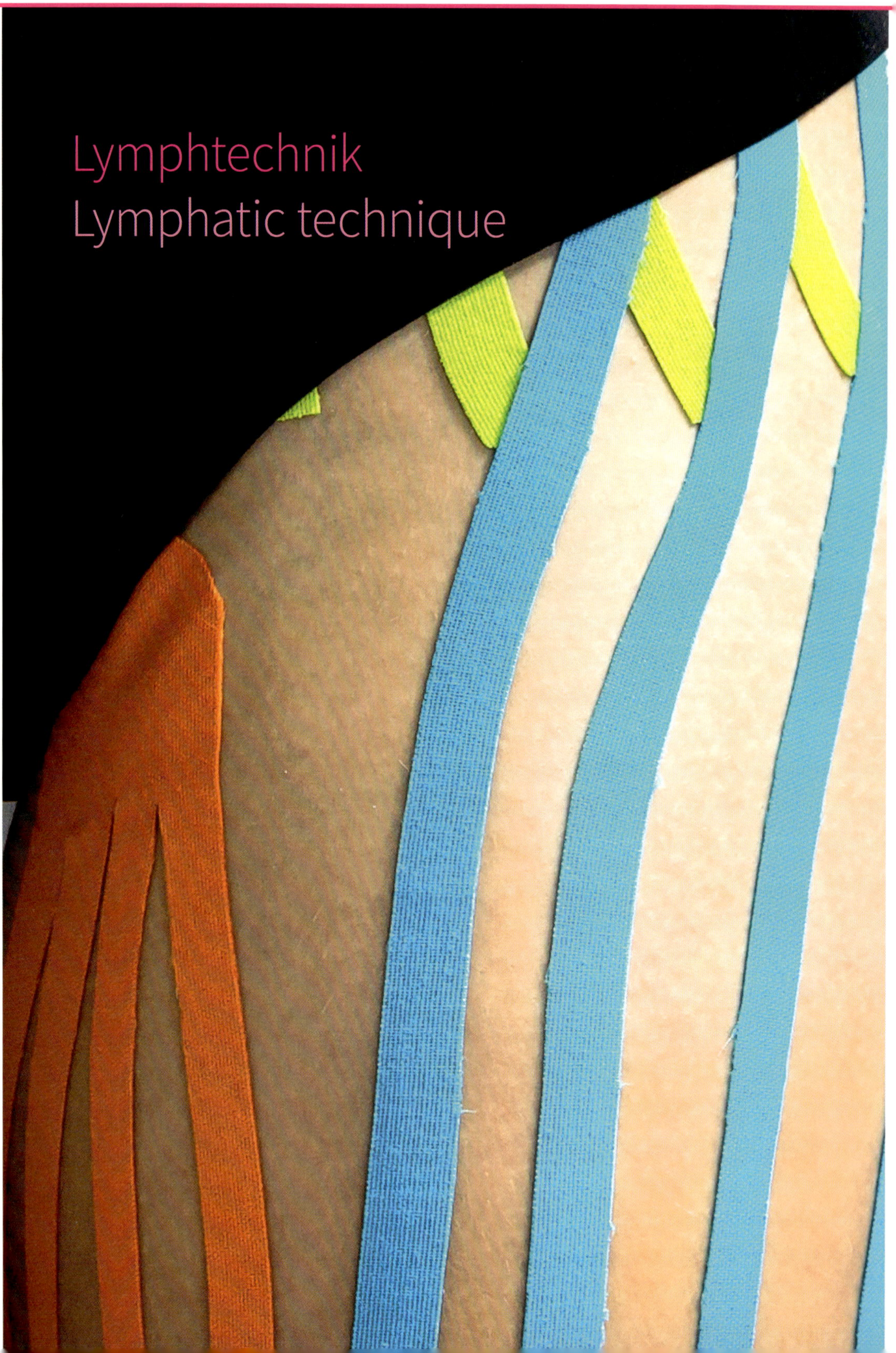

Wann wird diese Technik angewendet?

- Lymphatische Entstauung
- Entstaut das Gewebe
- Abtransport von Hämatomen
- Kann Adhäsionen (Verklebungen) im Gewebe weich massieren

Kleberichtung

An Armen und Beinen Basis des Tapes immer von den Lymphknoten in die Peripherie (von oben nach unten oder proximal nach distal)

When is this technique used?

- Lymphatic decongestion
- Tissue decongestion
- Drainage of haematomas
- Gentle massage of tissue adhesions

Direction of application

On the arms and legs, the base of the tape always being applied from the lymph nodes towards the periphery (in a downward or proximal to distal direction)

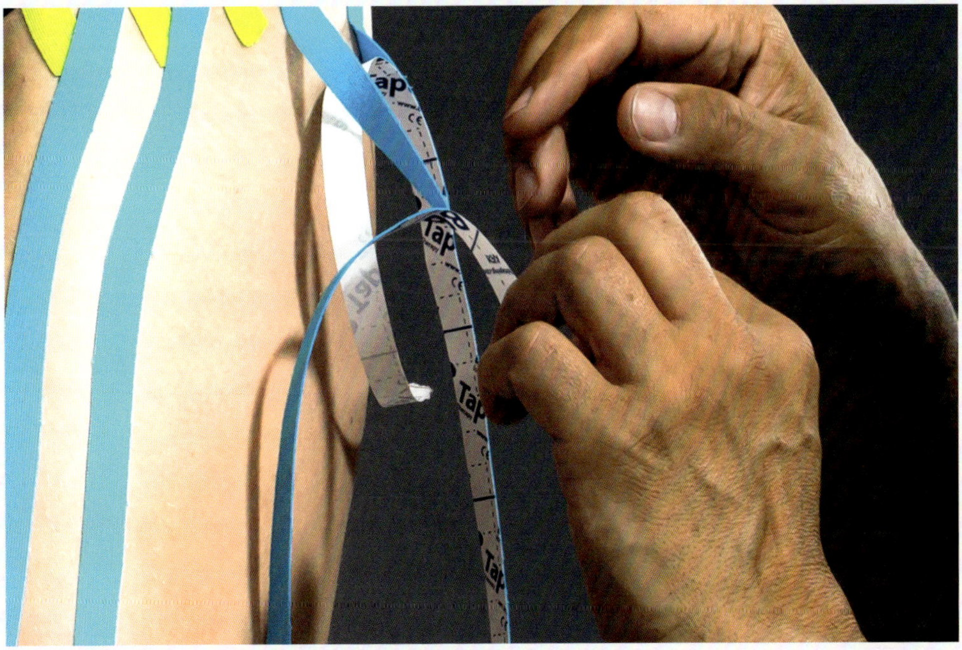

LYMPHTECHNIK – So wird's gemacht!
LYMPHATIC TECHNIQUE – That's how it's done!

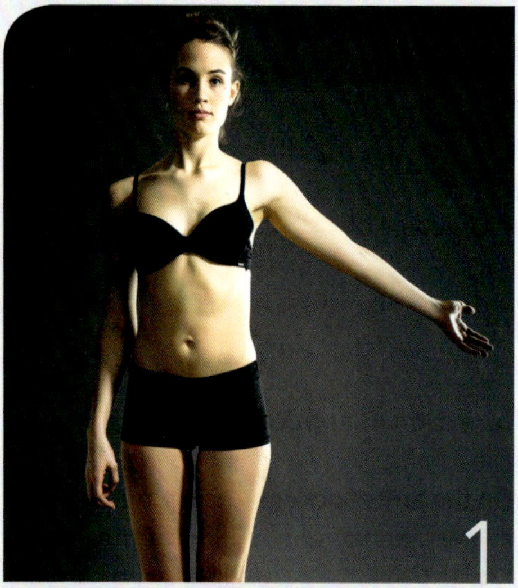

1

Haut und Muskeln so gut es geht vor dem Aufkleben vordehnen

Pre-stretch the skin and muscles as much as possible prior to affixing the tape

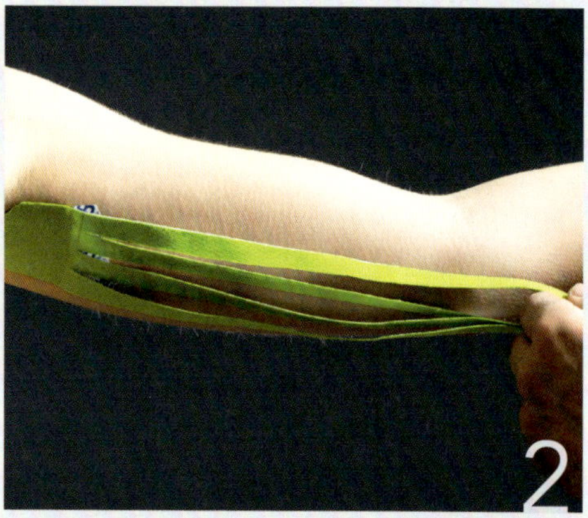

2

Tape in 4 Streifen schneiden. Den 1. Schnitt in der Mitte des Tapes, dann die beiden schmalen Zügel wieder halbieren. Tapebasis immer in Abflussrichtung der Lymphe kleben (körpernah)

Cut the tape into 4 strips Make the 1st cut in the centre of the tape and then halve the two narrow tails. Always affix the tape base in the direction of lymphatic drainage (proximally)

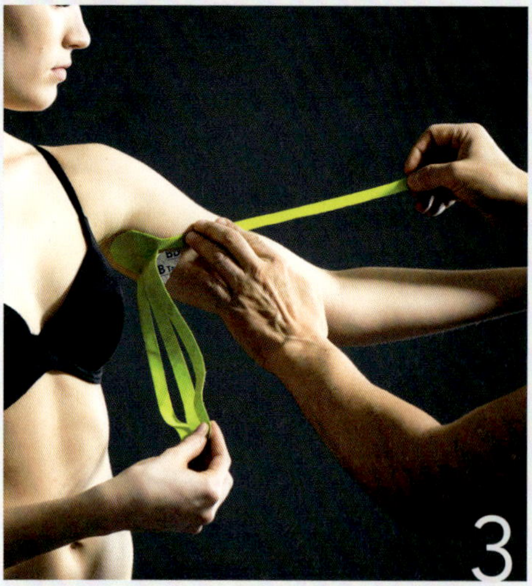

3

Tapezügel mit leichtem Zug max. 5 % aufkleben

Affix the tape tails with a slight stretch of 5% maximum

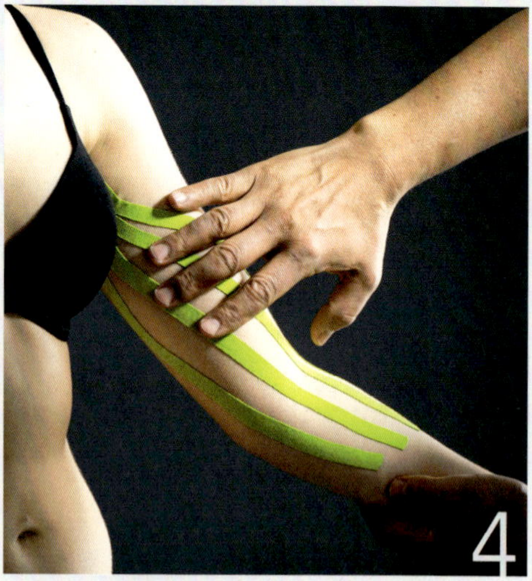

4

Tape anreiben

Rub down the tape

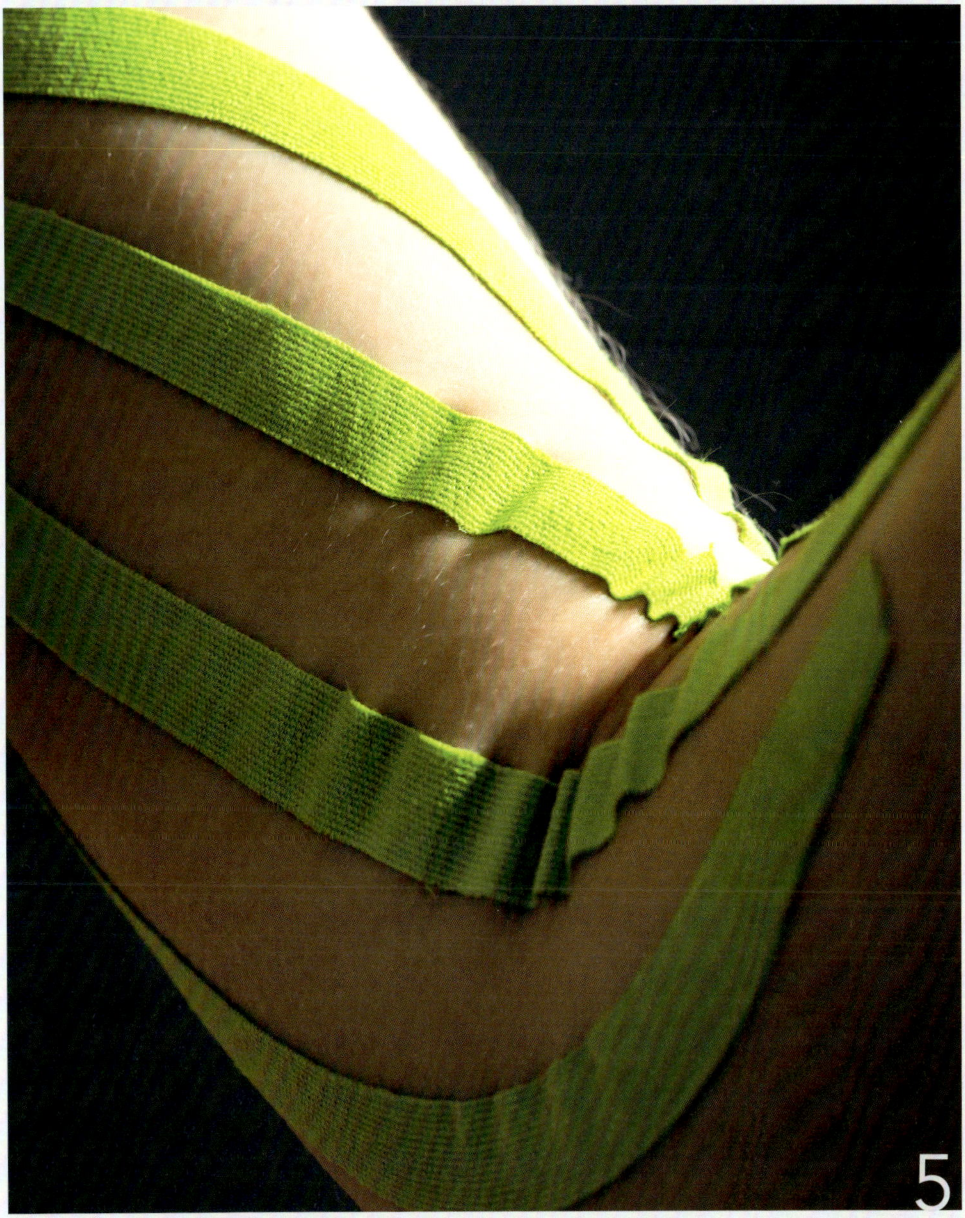

Effekt: Tape hebt die Haut an und aktiviert die Lymphmotorik

Effect: the tape lifts the skin and activates the lymphatic system

Faszientechnik
Fascia technique

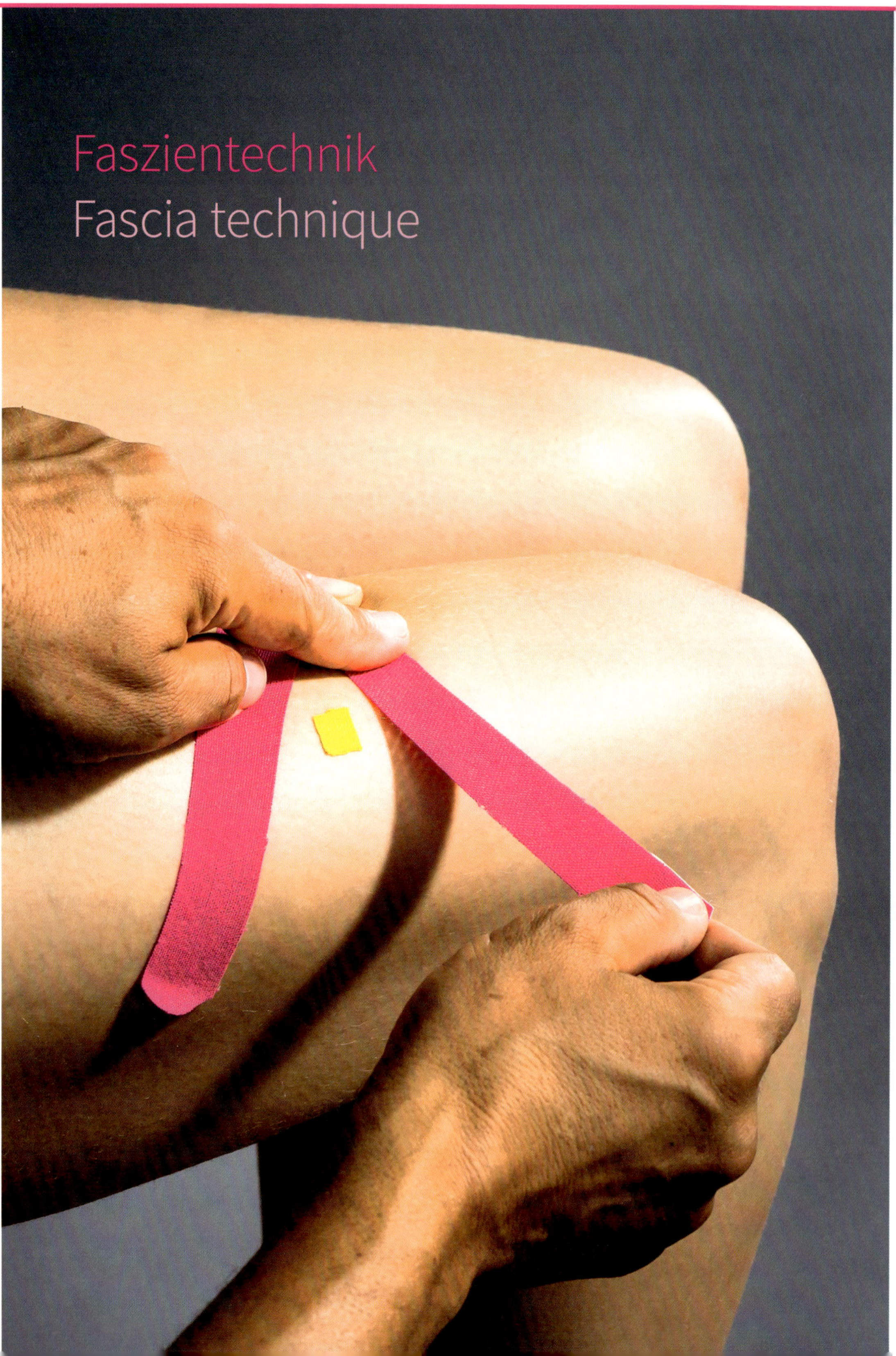

Wann wird diese Technik angewendet?

- Zum Lösen von Verklebungen im Gewebe

When is this technique used?

- To release tissue adhesions

Wirkung

- Schmerzentlastung
- Bessere Beweglichkeit der Gelenke

Effect

- Pain relief
- Better joint mobility

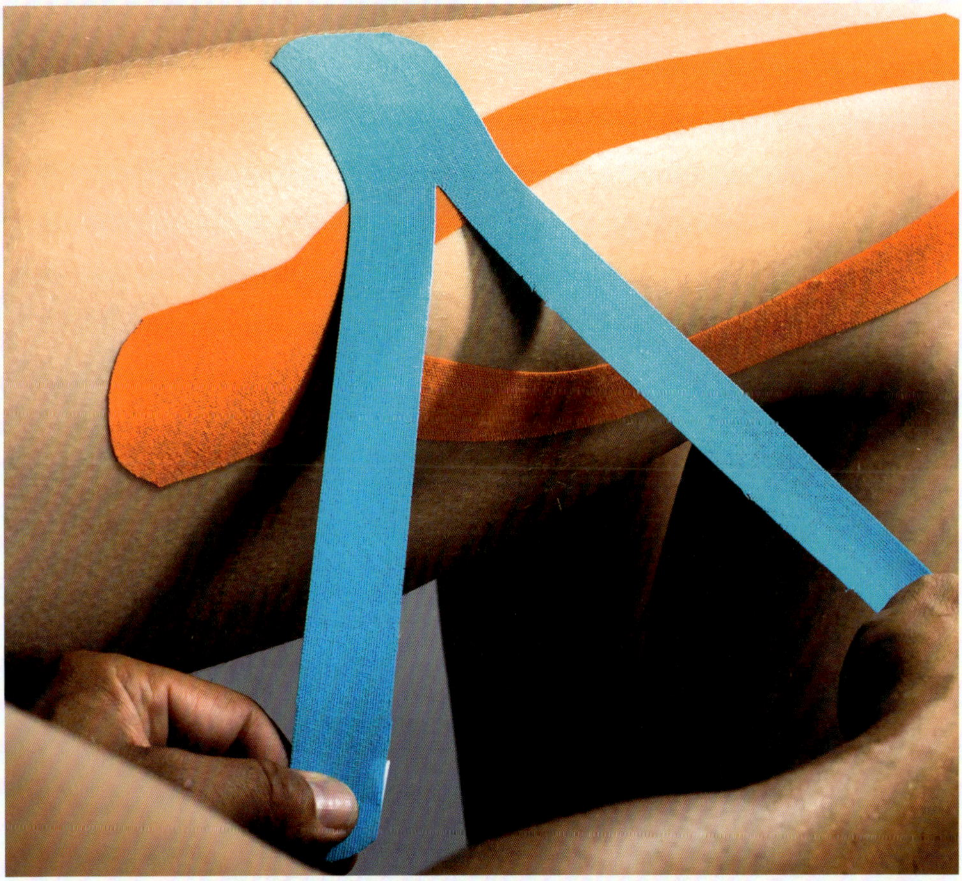

FASZIENTECHNIK – So wird's gemacht!
FASCIA TECHNIQUE – That's how it's done!

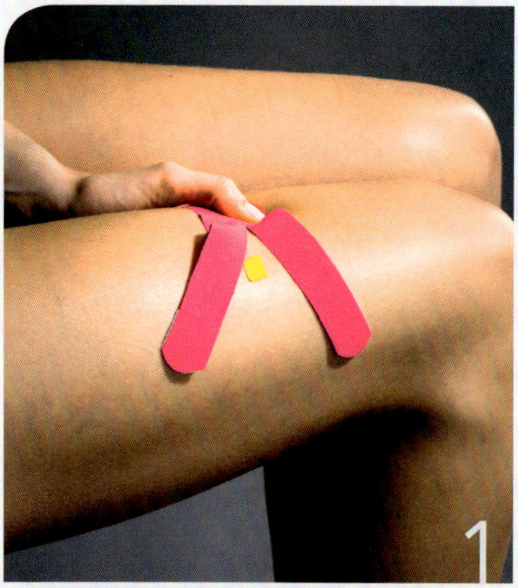

Tape zum Y schneiden und um Schmerzstelle herumlegen

Cut tape into a Y shape and place around the painful area

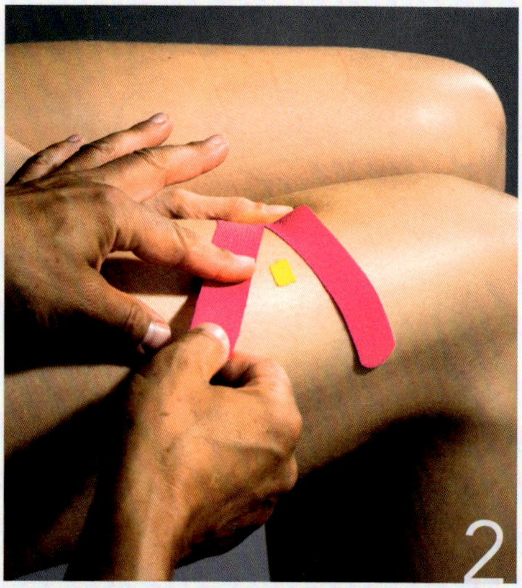

Tapebasis mit Finger auf Zug halten

Keep tape base stretched using the fingers

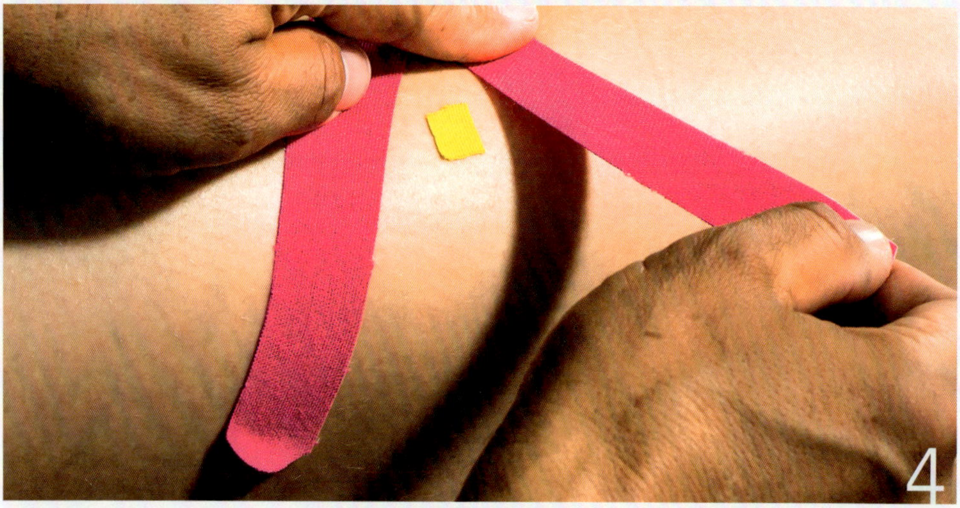

Tapezügel mit leichtem Zug ca. 20 % aufkleben

Affix the tape tails with a slight stretch of about 20%

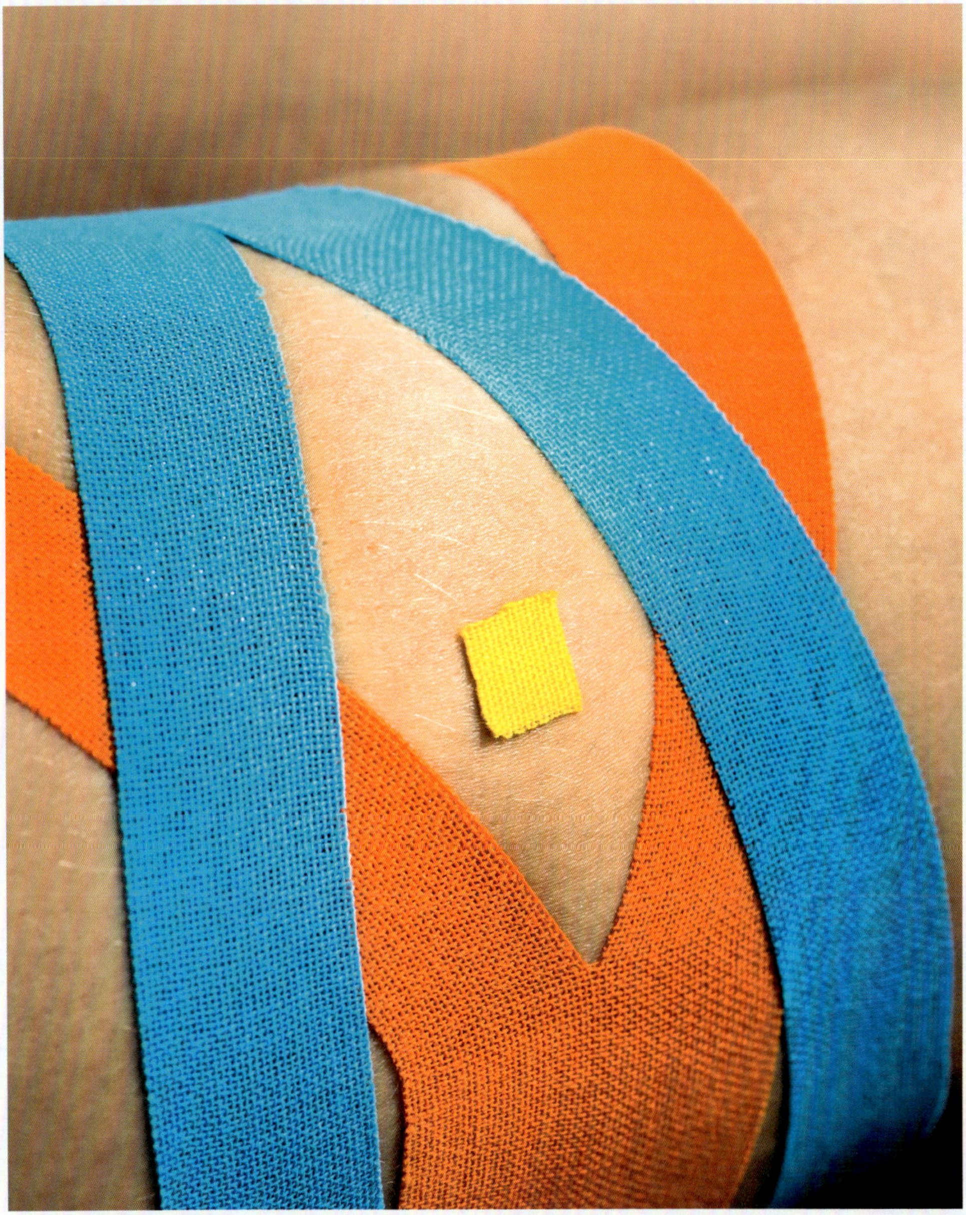

Mechanische Technik (Korrekturtechnik)

Mechanical technique (corrective technique)

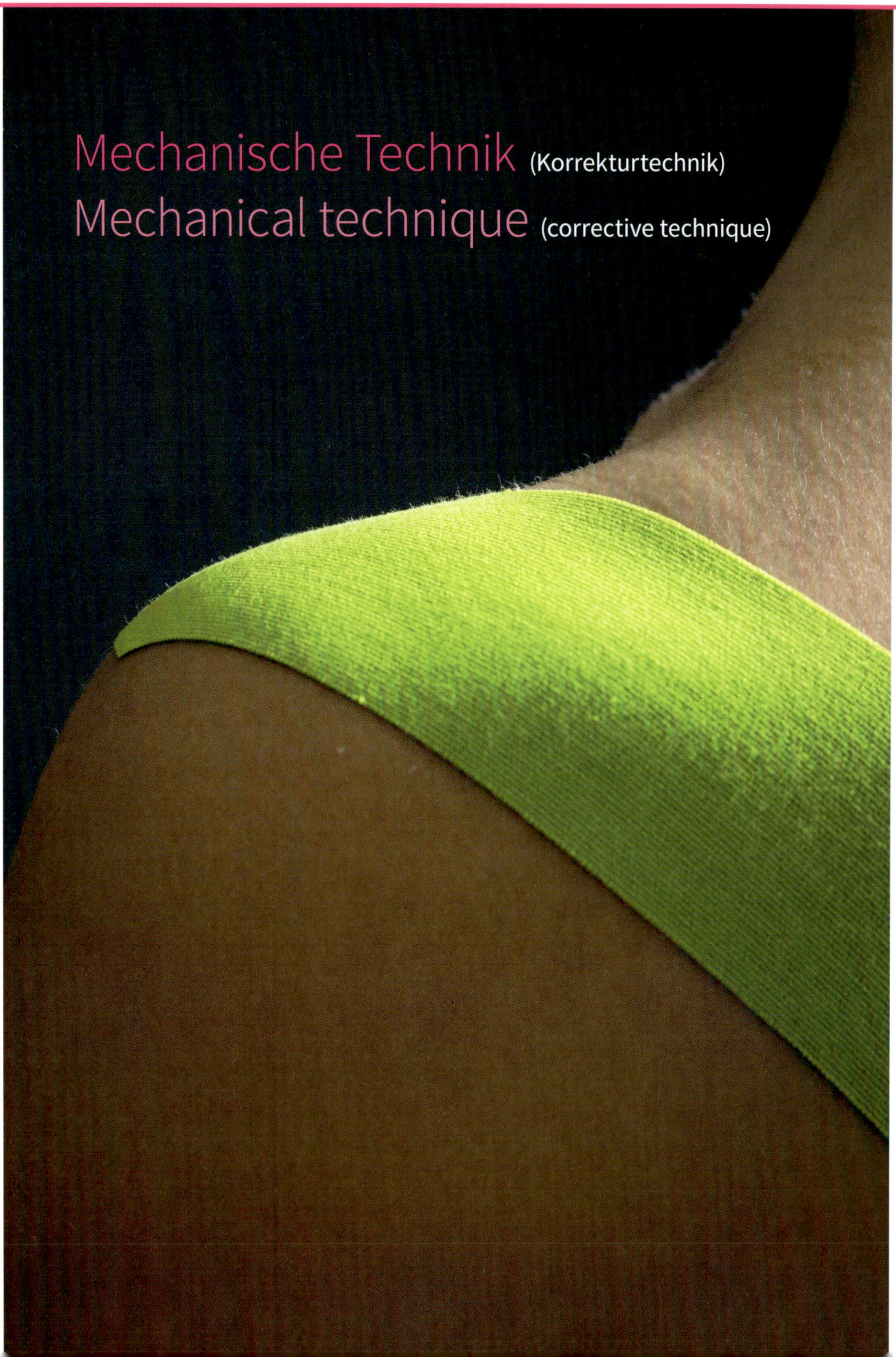

Wann wird diese Technik angewendet?

- Stabilisierung von Gelenken (Sprunggelenk, Schulter, Knie und Handgelenk)
- Korrektur von Fehlhaltungen
- Korrektur von Fußfehlstellungen (Knick-, Senk-, Spreizfuß)

Technik

- siehe Indikationen

When is this technique used?

- Joint stabilisation (ankle, shoulder, knee and wrist)
- Correction of poor posture
- Correction of foot misalignment (skewfoot, flat foot, splayfoot)

Technique

- see indications

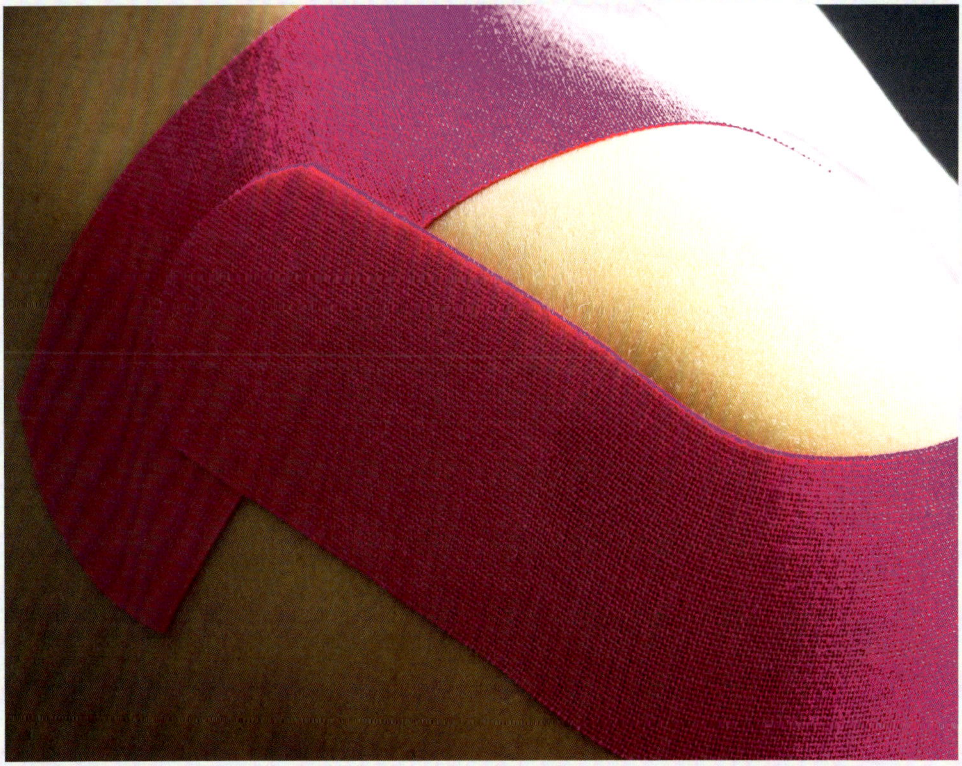

MECHANISCHE TECHNIK – So wird's gemacht!
MECHANICAL TECHNIQUE – That's how it's done!

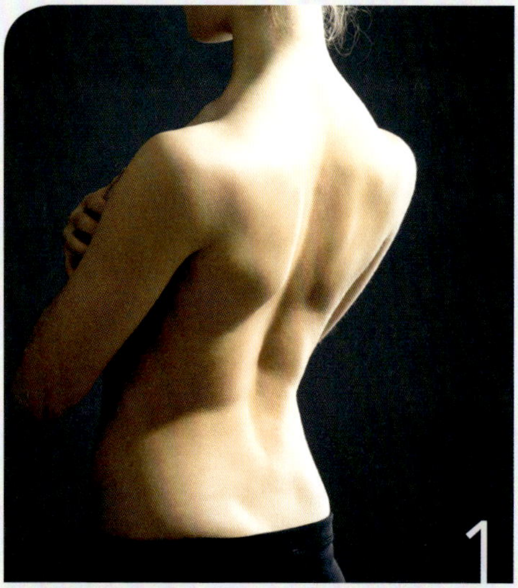

Überkorrigierte Haltung

Overcorrected posture

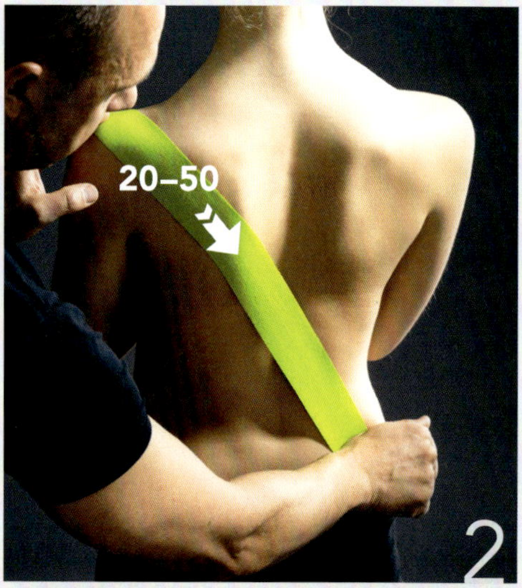

Tape mit leichtem Zug aufkleben

Affix the tape with a slight stretch

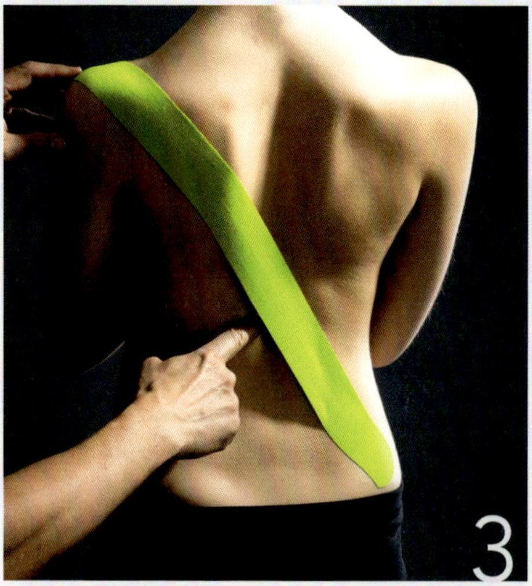

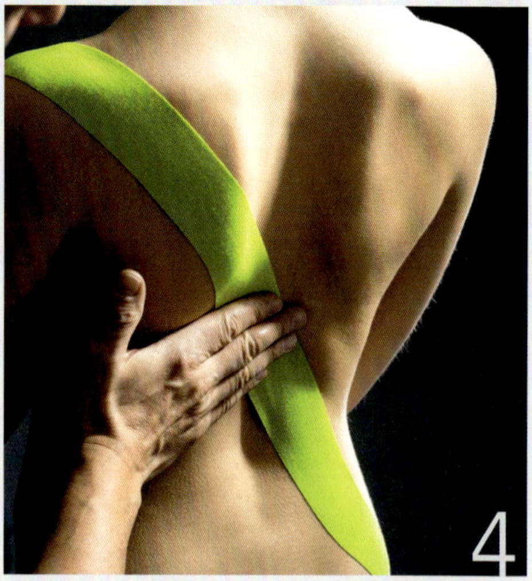

Körper beugen und entlasten, das Tape klebt sich nun von alleine faltenfei auf dem Körper auf. Zum Schluss das Tape anreiben

Bend and relax the body; the tape will now adhere to the body by itself without wrinkling. Finally, rub down the tape

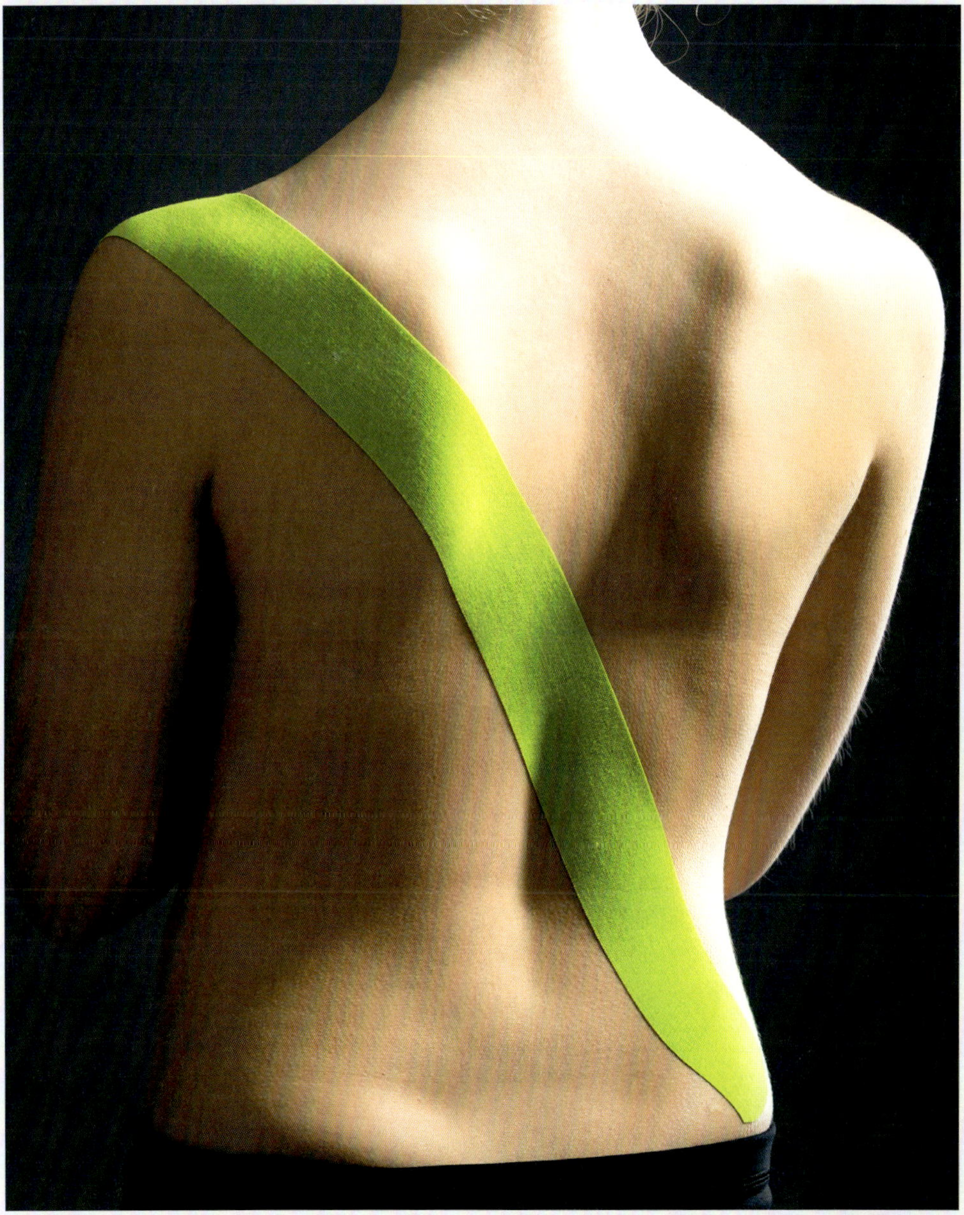

Gitterpflaster
Cross-tapes

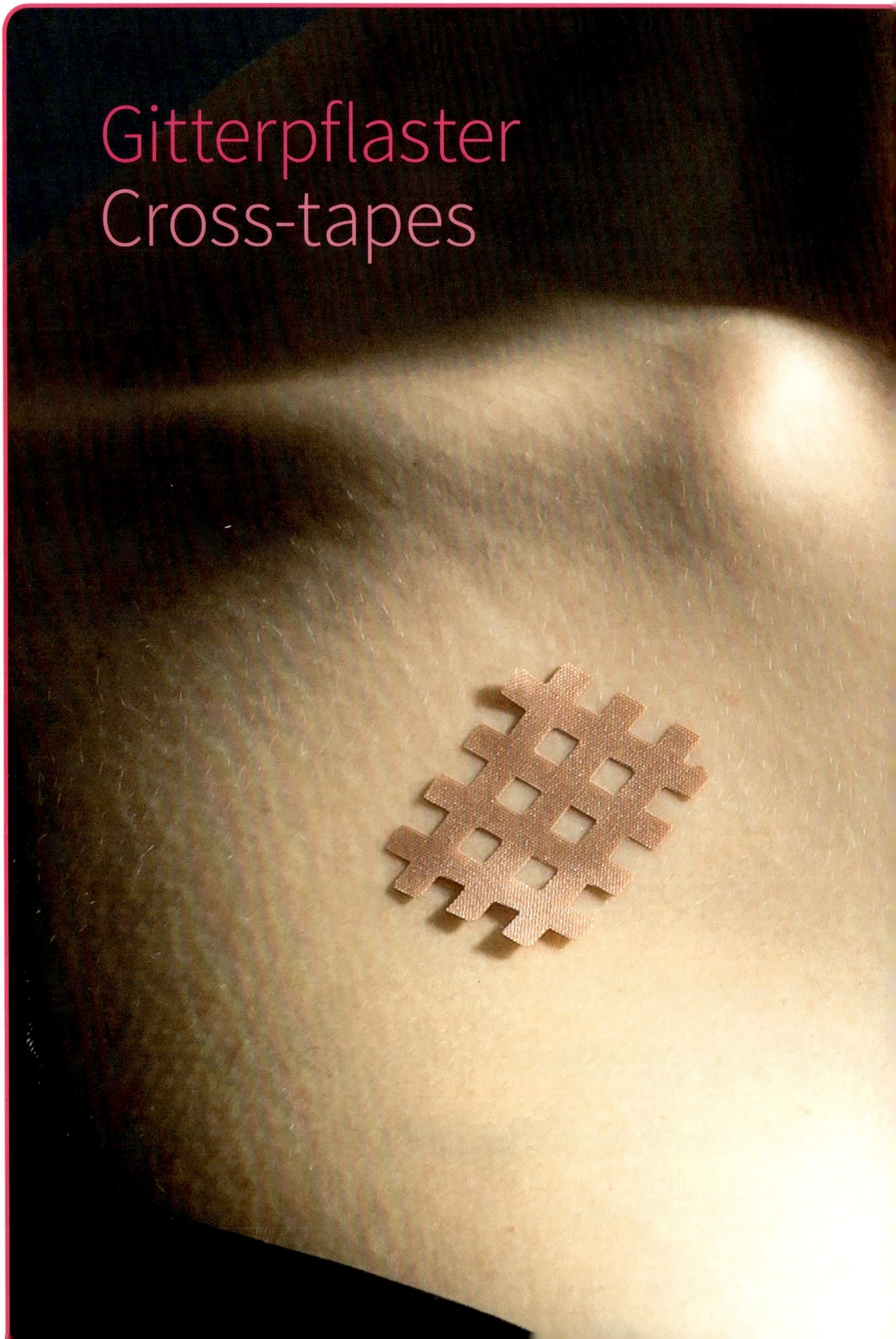

Sanfte Reize – Große Wirkung

Gitterpflaster sind kleine unelastische Pflaster ohne Wirkstoffe. Ihre außerordentliche Wirkung erzielen sie über die Entlastung der Hautoberfläche in den kleinen Quadraten. In Asien eine sehr bekannte Methode.

Gentle stimuli – Big effect

Cross-tapes are small inelastic patches not containing any active substances. They achieve their extraordinary effect by decompressing the skin's surface in the small squares. A very well-known method in Asia.

Anwendungsgebiete
Indications

- Zur Wirkungsverstärkung der kinesiologischen Tapeverbände
- Zur Aktivierung der körpereigenen Reperaturmechanismen
- Zur Schmerzreduktion
- Zur Schwellungsreduktion
- Als Alternative zur Akupunkturnadel
- Zur Behandlung von Reflexzonen
- Zur Unterstützung des Körpers in der Genesung bei Erkältungskrankheiten
- Zur Behandlung von gestörten und schmerzhaften Muskeln, Sehnen, Bändern und Gelenken
- Zur Narbenbehandlung
- Bei Kopfschmerzen

- To enhance the effect of kinesiology tape dressings
- To activate the body's natural repair mechanisms
- To reduce pain
- To reduce swelling
- As an alternative to acupuncture needles
- To treat reflex zones
- To assist the body's recovery from colds
- To treat injured and painful muscles, tendons, ligaments and joints
- To treat scars
- To treat headaches

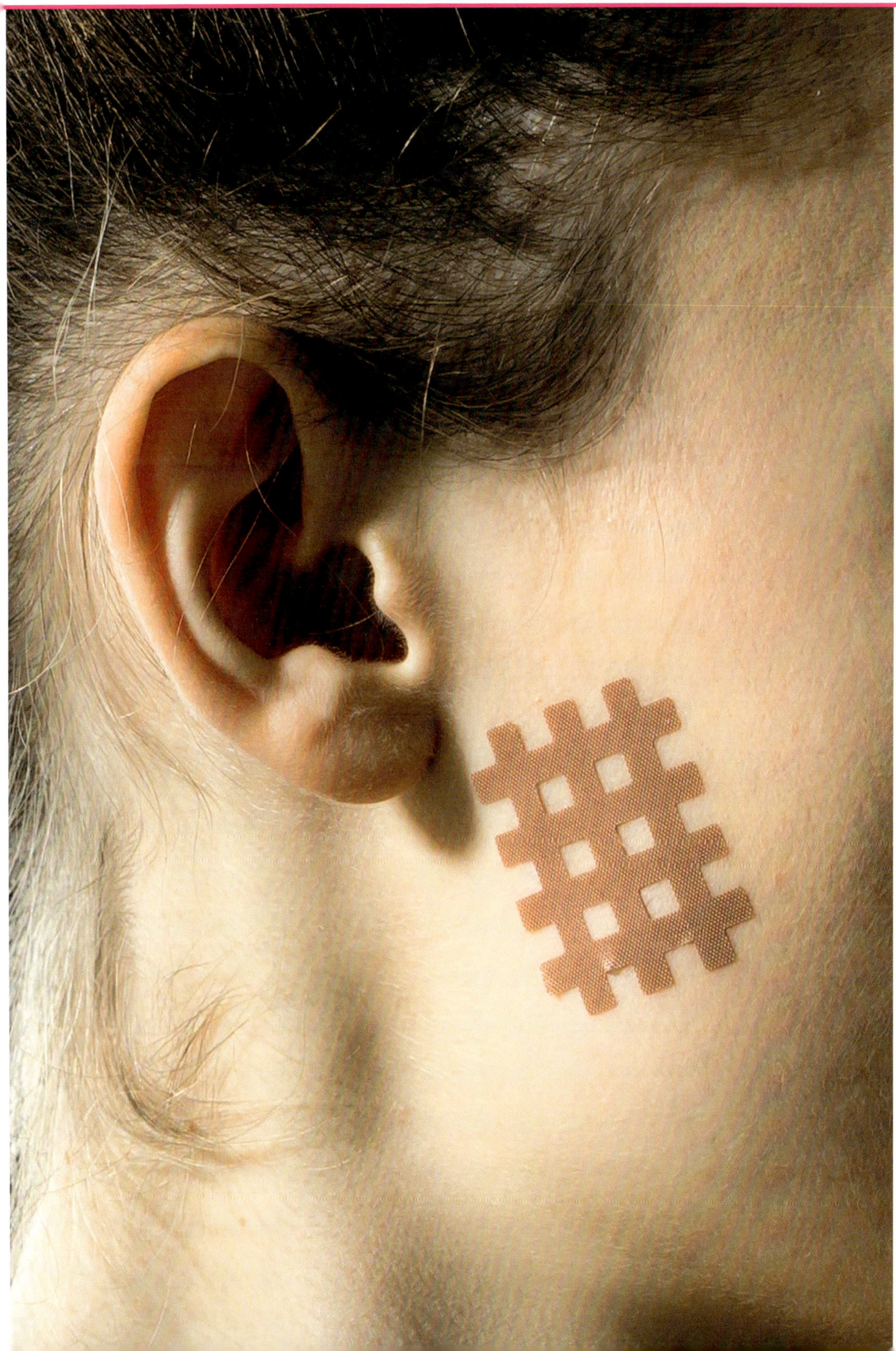

Die Gitterpflastermethode

Gesund ohne Wirkstoffe

„In Asien altbewährt, bei uns neu entdeckt"

Gitterpflaster können bei einer Vielzahl von Beschwerden eingesetzt werden:

Schmerzen:

- Rücken
- Nacken
- Kopf
- Magen
- Gelenke
- Ohren

Entzündungen:

- Hals
- Nasennebenhöhlen
- Haut

Und das Besondere der Gitterpflastermethode: Die Gitterpflaster kann jeder selbst schnell und einfach anwenden.

Zusätzliche Informationen für Ärzte und Therapeuten

Bereichern Sie Ihr Versorgungsrepertoire. In Asien ist die Gitterpflastermethode in Kombination mit dem kinesiologischen Tapen seit Jahren bewährt.

Bieten auch Sie Ihren Patienten diese geniale Methode an! Und das ohne zusätzliche Medikamente und Inhaltsstoffe.

Die Gitterpflaster direkt auf die Schmerzpunkte und auf die in der Literatur (Die Heilkraft der Gitterpflaster & Mein Magisches Pflaster) beschriebenen Akupunktur- und Reflexpunkte kleben. Oftmals schon nach kurzer Zeit können Ihre Patienten die schmerzlindernde Wirkung spüren.

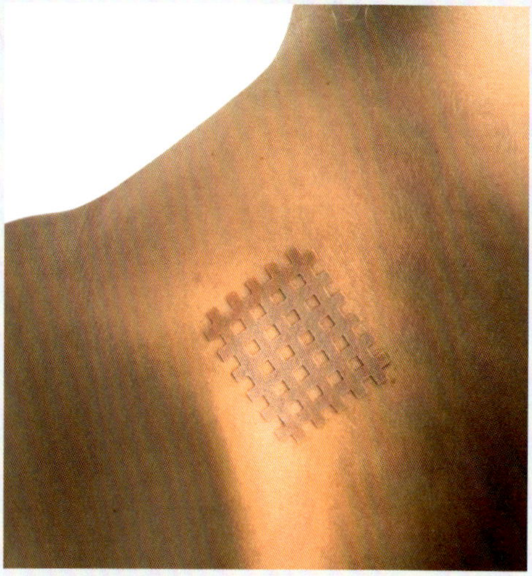

The cross-tape method

Healthy without active substances

"Long-established in Asia, newly discovered by us"

Cross-tapes can be used for many types of discomfort:

Pain:

- Back
- Neck
- Head
- Stomach
- Joints
- Ears

Additional information for doctors and therapists

Enhance your treatment repertoire. In Asia, the cross-tape method has been used successfully for years in combination with kinesiology tapes.

Why not offer your patients this ingenious method yourself! Without additional medicines and ingredients, to boot.

Affix the cross-tape directly to the painful spots and to the acupuncture and reflex points described in the literature (The Healing Power of lattice tapes & My magic lattice tape). Your patients will often be able to feel the pain-relieving effect after only a short time.

Inflammation:

- Throat
- Paranasal sinuses
- Skin

What makes the cross-tape method special is that anyone can use cross-tape quickly and easily.

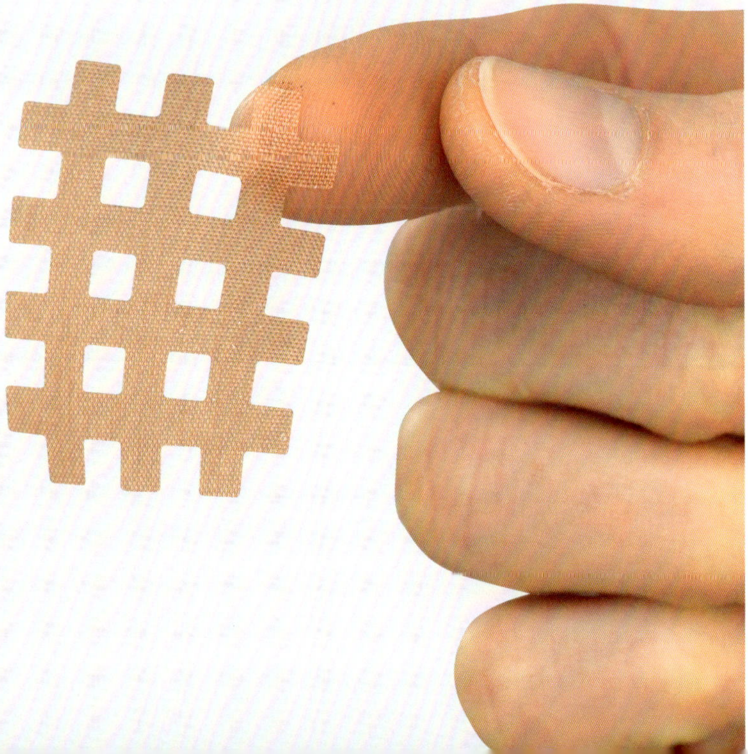

Das Wirkprinzip

Entlastungsreize über die Hautoberfläche

Blockaden und Schmerzen, die durch Druck und Belastung ausgelöst werden, können durch Entlastung behoben werden.

Die Verbindung unseres Körpers zur Außenwelt ist die Haut. Sie ist ein komplexes Organ, das mit tausenden von Fühlern (Rezeptoren) ausgestattet ist. Dadurch wird uns signalisiert, was außerhalb des Körpers passiert (Kälte, Wärme, Druck…), und auch, wie es dem Körper im Inneren geht (Stress, Nervosität, Angst…).

Die Haut reagiert sichtbar mit Rötungen, Gänsehaut, Schwitzen, Entzündungen u.ä. Das kennen wir alle und erleben es tagtäglich. Das bedeutet, dass die Haut auch in der Lage ist, tief im Inneren des Körpers mithilfe der Rezeptoren Reaktionen hervorzurufen.

Positive Einflüsse

Positive Einflüsse (Entlastungsreize) auf die Haut, auch durch die Gitterpflaster, werden von uns als angenehm und wohltuend empfunden.

Wir können entspannen, loslassen, genießen; die Blockaden lösen sich. Es geht uns zunehmend besser.

Was passiert unter den Gittern?

Wenn Sie ein Gitterpflaster aufkleben, wird die Haut in den einzelnen Feldern innerhalb der Gitterstruktur bei der kleinsten Bewegung durch ein leichtes Anheben entlastet. Diese Mikroentlastung aktiviert die Hautsensoren und führt zu einer Vielzahl von Reaktionen im Körper.

Wir empfinden:

- weniger Schmerzen;
- Entzündungen heilen schneller ab;
- Blockaden lösen sich;
- Muskelverspannungen werden gelockert;
- der Körper wird ins Gleichgewicht gebracht;
- die Mikrozirkulation wird angeregt (siehe Hautrötung auf der folgenden Darstellung).

Mode of action

Decompression stimuli over the skin's surface

Blockages and pain triggered by pressure and loading can be alleviated by decompression.

The skin is our body's connection with the outside world. It is a complex organ equipped with thousands of sensors (receptors). They alert us to what is happening outside the body (cold, heat, pressure, etc.) and also to how our bodies are feeling on the inside (stress, nervousness, anxiety, etc.).

The skin responds visibly with redness, goose bumps, sweating, inflammation, etc. We are all familiar with them and experience them on a daily basis. This means that the skin is also capable of triggering reactions deep inside the body with the aid of the receptors.

Positive influences

We find positive influences (decompression stimuli) on the skin, including those produced by cross-tapes, to be pleasant and beneficial.

We are able to relax, let go, experience enjoyment; the blockages release. We feel better and better.

What is happening underneath the cross-tapes?

When you affix a cross-tape, the skin in the individual squares inside the lattice structure is decompressed by lifting slightly in response to the smallest movement. This micro-decompression activates the sensors in the skin and causes the body to respond in a whole host of ways.

We experience:

- less pain;
- more rapid healing of inflammation;
- the release of blockages;
- a loosening of muscle tension;
- balancing of the body;
- stimulation of the microcirculation (see the skin redness on the following illustration).

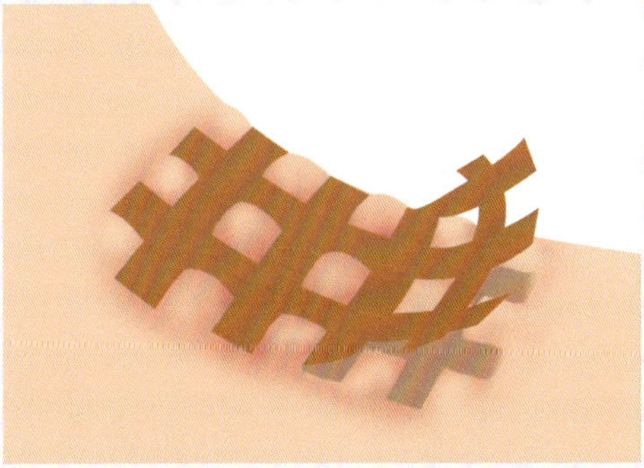

Wie werden die Gitter angewendet?
How are the cross-tapes used?

Wichtig ist, die richtigen Gitterpflaster zu nehmen

Nur die originalen und qualitativ hochwertigen Gitterpflaster (z. B. aus Korea) ziehen sich dank ihrer elektrostatischen Aufladung an die Schmerzpunkte heran, bieten eine sehr gute Klebkraft und eignen sich auch für Kinderhaut. Sie sind hautfreundlich und überzeugen mit ihrer sicheren Klebkraft (auch unter Einwirkung von Wasser). Die Gitterpflaster lassen sich schnell und unkompliziert nach den im Anwendungsbuch beschriebenen Anweisungen aufkleben.

Hinweis

Kleben Sie die Gitterpflaster nicht auf erkrankte, verletzte oder offene Hautstellen. Nach Symptomlinderung darf das Gitterpflaster abgenommen werden.

Weitere Informationen erhalten Sie unter:
www.gitterpflaster-okamed.de

It is important to use the correct cross-tapes

Due to their electrostatic charge, only the original, high-quality cross-tapes (e.g. from Korea) stimulate the painful spots, offer very good adhesive strength and are also suitable for children's skin. They are skin-friendly and adhere securely (including in contact with water). The cross-tapes can be affixed quickly and easily following the instructions in the manual.

Please note

Do not affix the cross-tapes to diseased, injured or broken skin. The cross-tape can be removed once the symptoms have been alleviated.

You will find further information at:
www.gitterpflaster-okamed.de

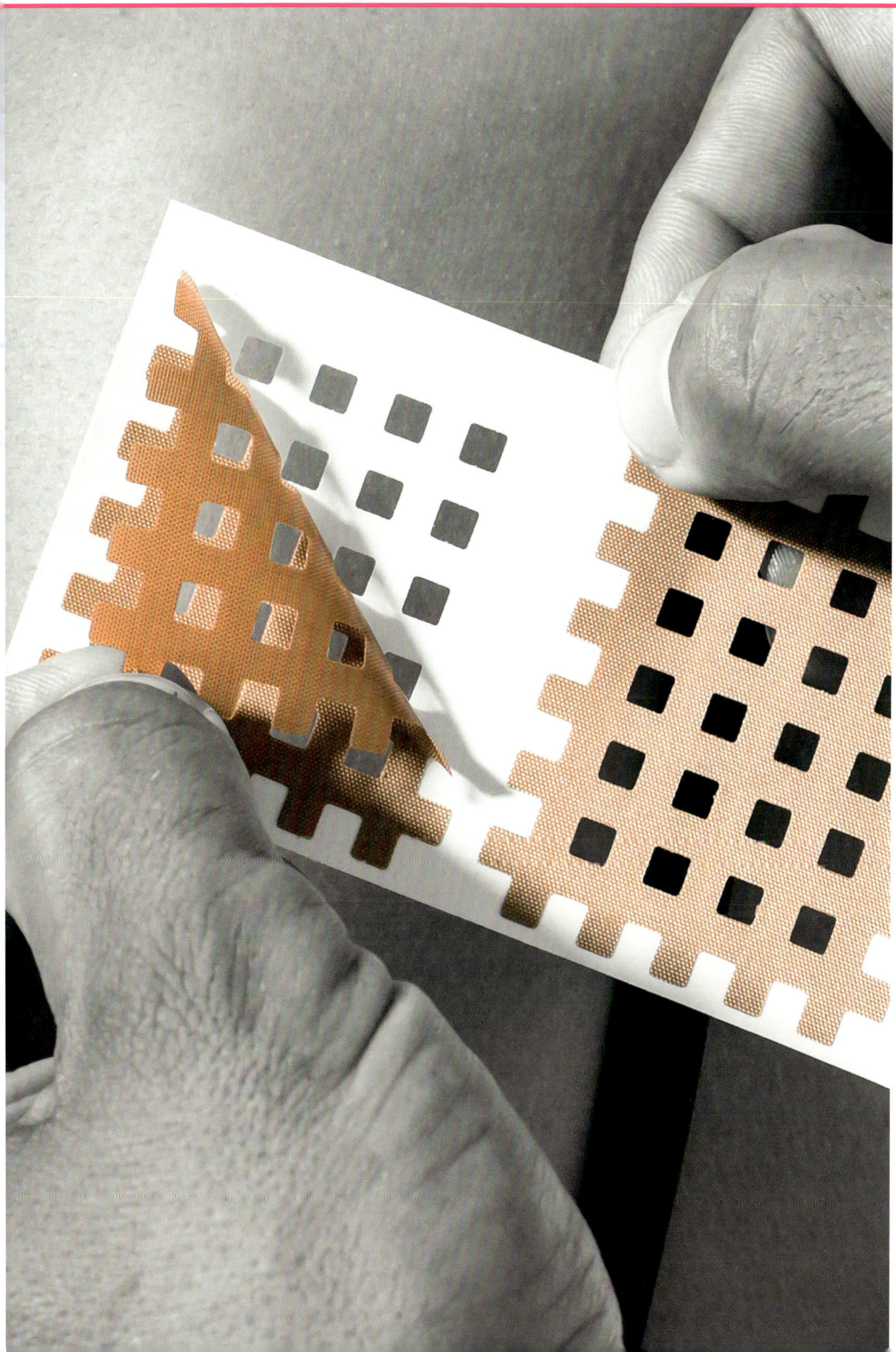

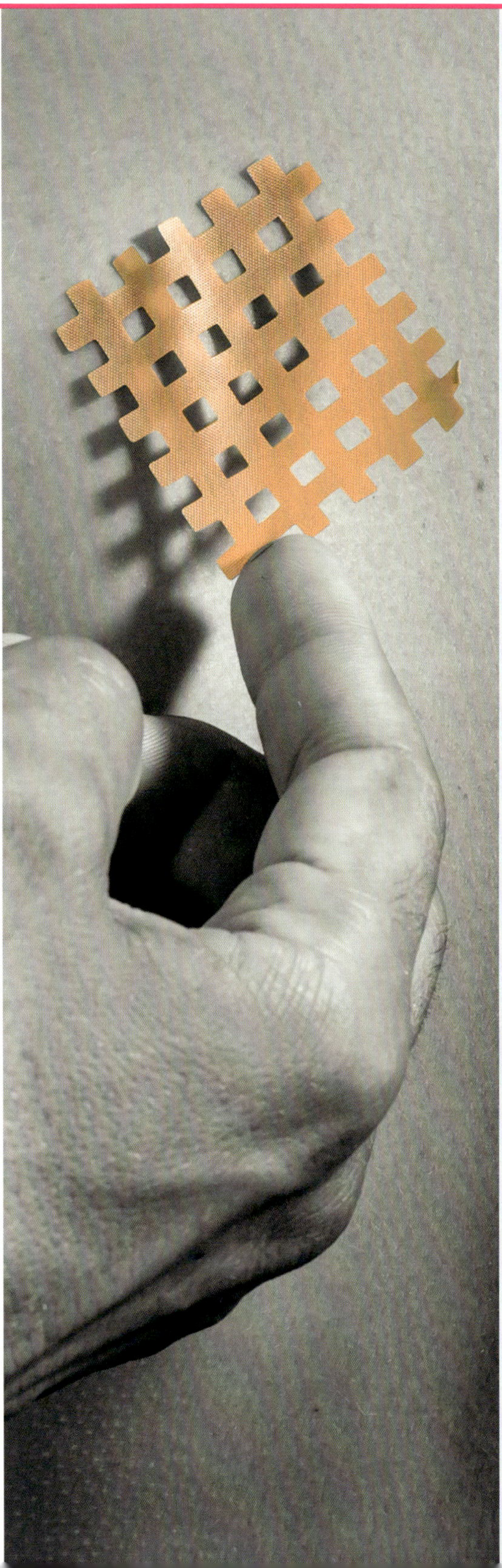

Anwendung in nur 2 Schritten!

1. Schritt

Zunächst kleben Sie die Gitter immer auf die schmerzenden Stellen am Körper.

2. Schritt

Da der Körper oftmals noch an anderen Stellen Blockaden aufweist, können weitere Gitter auf die für diese Beschwerden entsprechenden Akupunktur- und Reflexpunkte geklebt werden. Diese Punkte finden Sie für über 120 Beschwerdearten in den Anwendungsbüchern des international anerkannten Medical Trainers und Buchautors Olaf Kandt.

Applied in just 2 steps!

Step 1

First, always affix the cross-tape to the painful areas of the body.

Step 2

As the body often also has blockages in other areas, further cross-tapes can be affixed to the acupuncture and reflex points corresponding to this discomfort. You can find these points for over 120 types of discomfort in the instruction manuals of the internationally recognised medical trainer and book author, Olaf Kandt.

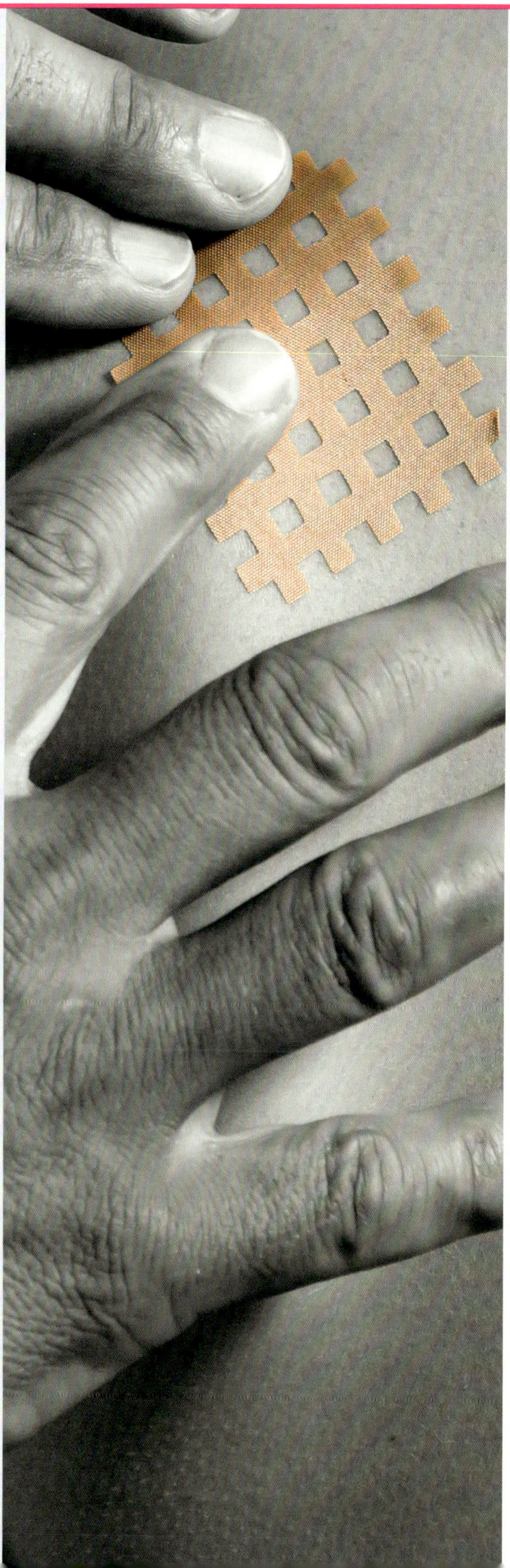

Buchempfehlung

Das Anwendungsbuch für Erwachsene „Die Heilkraft der Gitterpflaster“

Auf 400 Seiten erklärt Olaf Kandt – mit vielen, aussagekräftigen Abbildungen – an über 100 Krankheitsbildern die korrekte Platzierung der Gitterpflaster.

Recommended reading

Instruction manual for adults: “The Healing Power of lattice tapes”

In 400 pages, Olaf Kandt explains the correct cross-tape positioning for over 100 conditions, with lots of informative pictures.

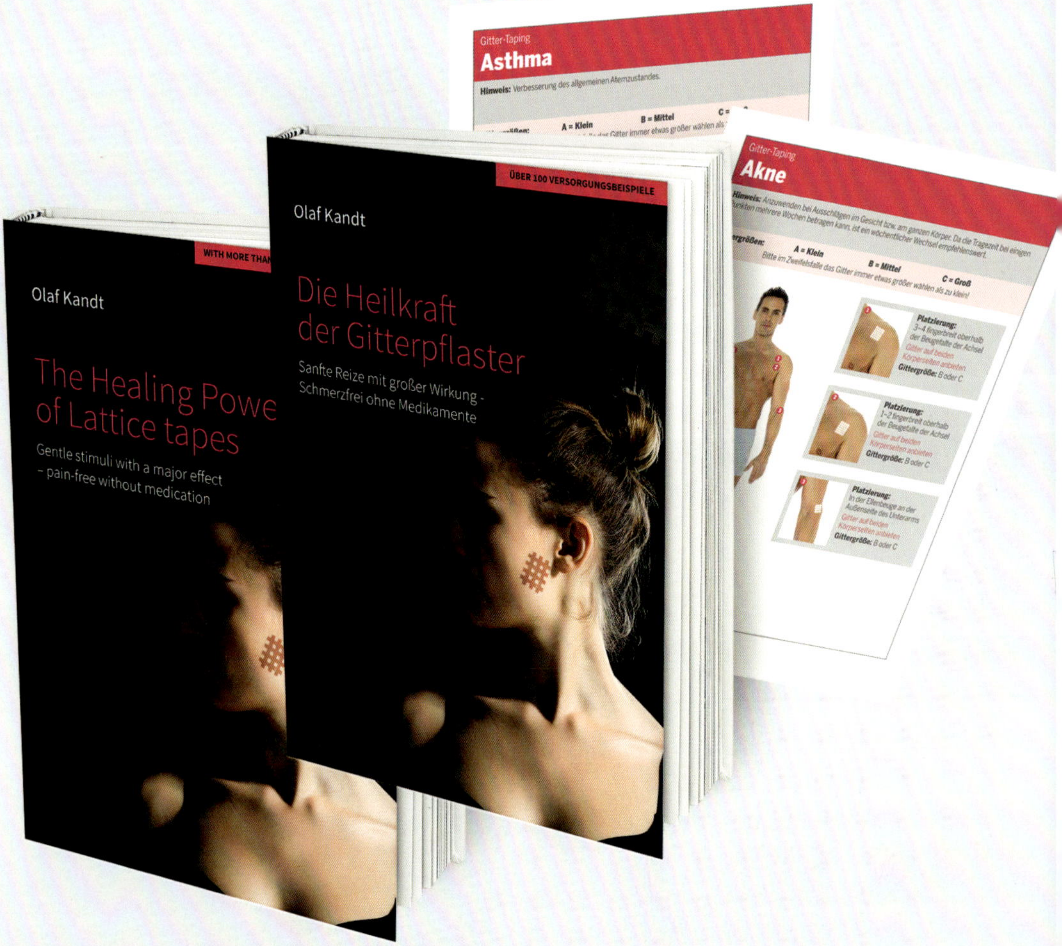

Das Anwendungsbuch für Kinder „Mein Magisches Pflaster“

Ebenfalls von Olaf Kandt: Hier wird auf 200 Seiten die Platzierung der Gitterpflaster bei 35 kindertypischen Beschwerdebildern erklärt. Ein kindgerechtes Anwendungsbuch mit vielen bunten Seiten für die Kinder und wenig Text, damit Eltern ihre Kinder schnell und effektiv versorgen können.

Instruction manual for children: “My magic lattice tape”

Also by Olaf Kandt: cross-tape positioning for 35 typical childhood conditions is explained in 200 pages. A child-oriented instruction manual with lots of colourful pages for children and little text so that parents can treat their children quickly and effectively.

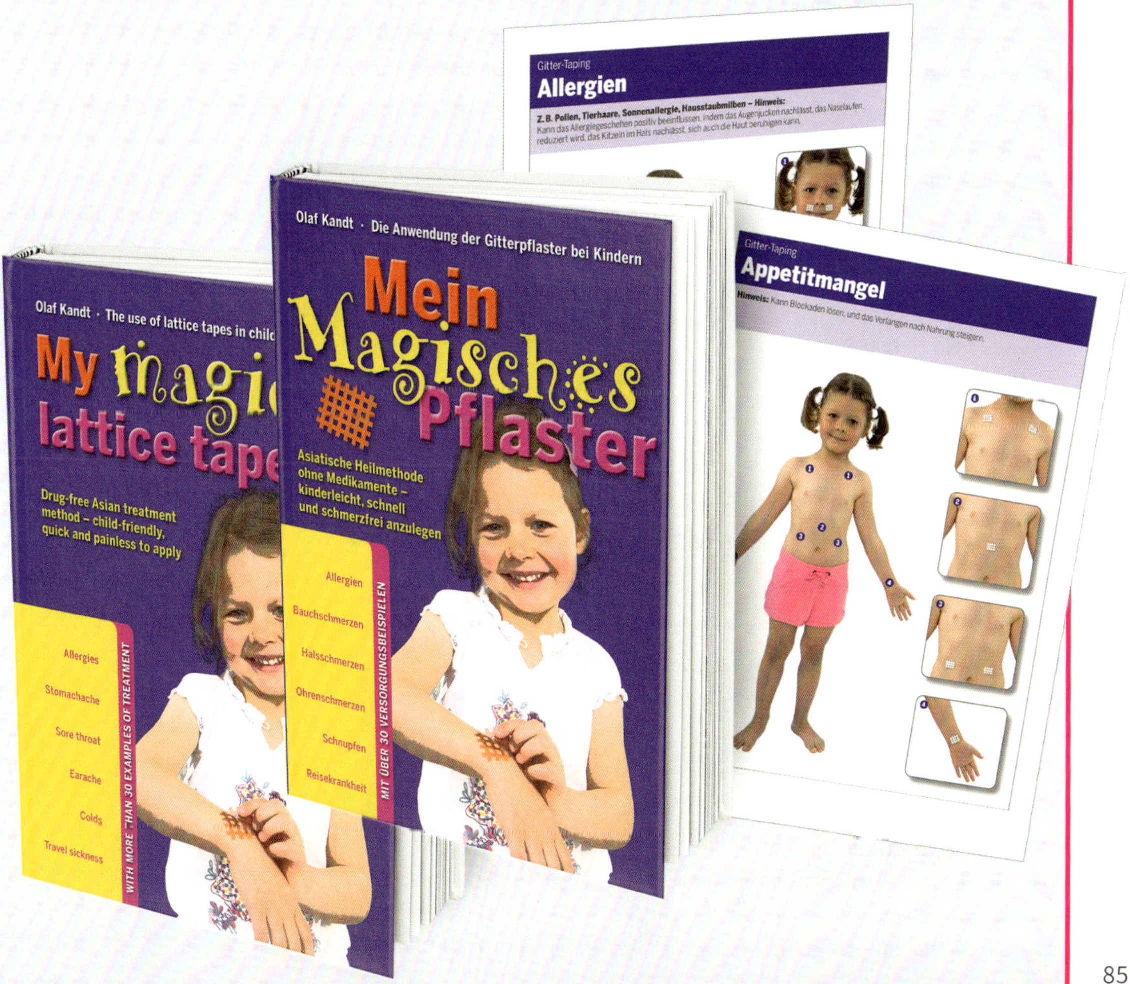

Indikationen
Indications

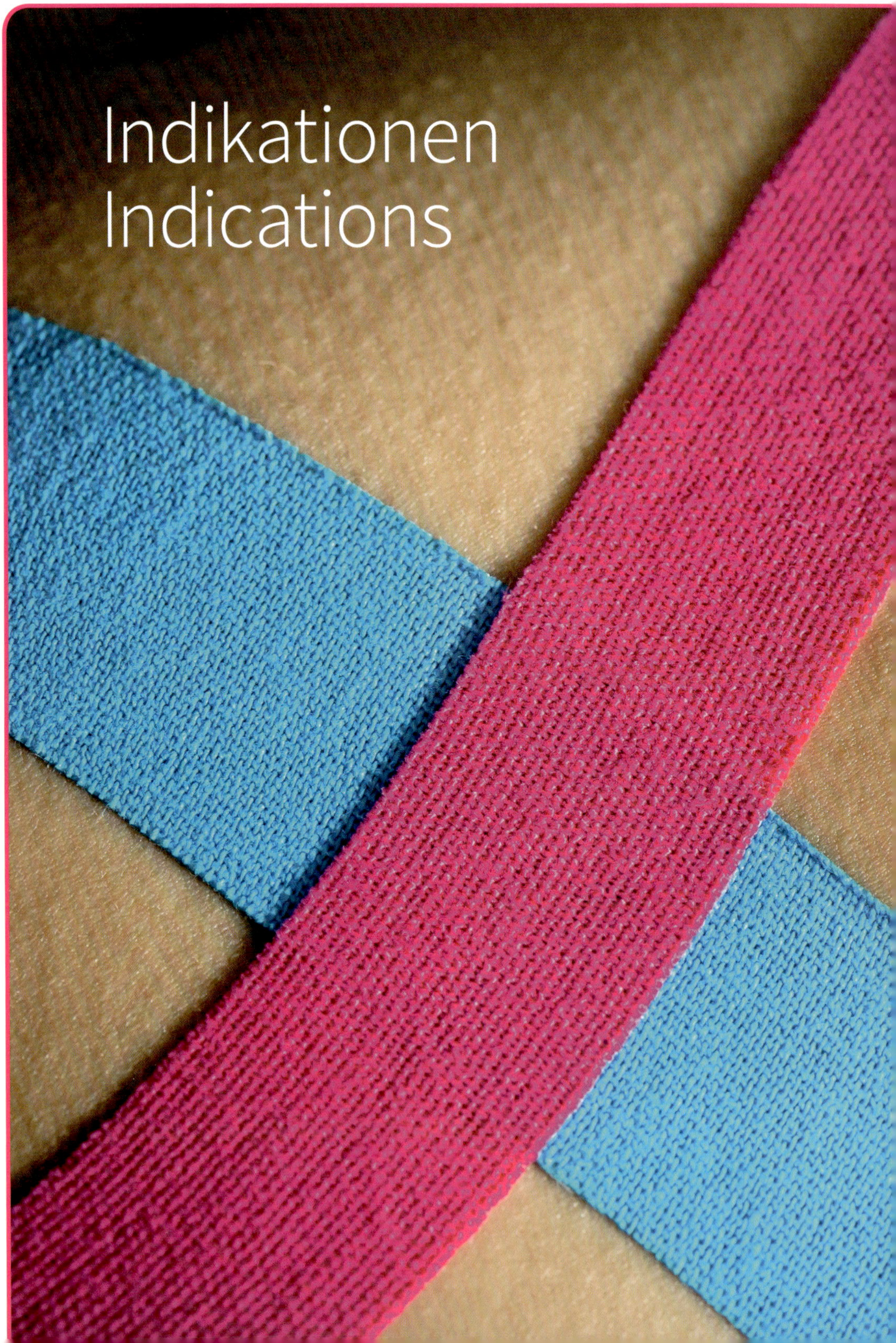

Inhalt – Contents

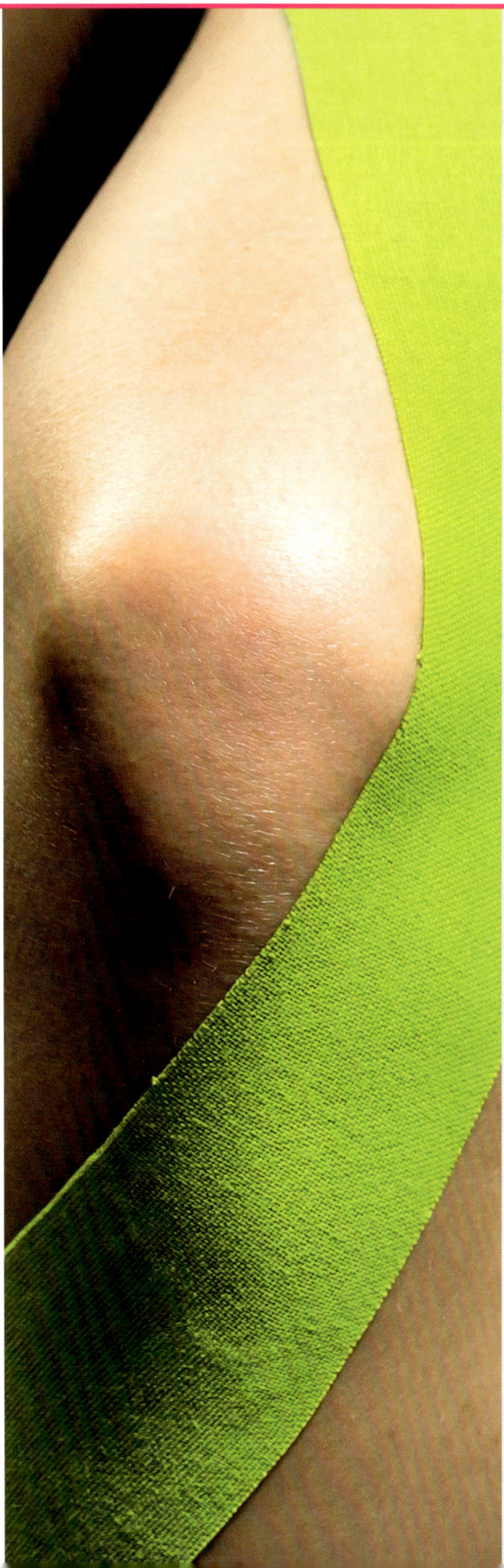

Tipp zur Vorgehensweise

Erst die Basistapes, wie beschrieben, kleben und 1–2 Tage abwarten. Je nachdem, wie sich dann noch die Beschwerden bemerkbar machen, können dann die optionalen Tapezügel zusätzlich aufgeklebt.

So kann die Tapeversorgung individuell den Beschwerden angepasst werden. Nach ca. 1 Woche Tragezeit sollte bei der neuen Tapeanlage der letzte Zügel nicht mehr aufgeklebt werden. Sollten mehrere Tapezügel aufgeklebt worden sein, bitte Woche für Woche immer den letzten Tape nicht mehr aufkleben bis kein Tape mehr notwendig ist. Die Tapeanlage darf je nach Beschwerden 4–6 mal angewendet werden (mit wöchentlichem Tapewechsel).

Länge der Tapes immer genauso abmessen wie auf den Bildern ersichtlich.

Basis Tape*:* Dieser Tapezügel sollte immer angelegt werden.

Tape optional: Bei Bedarf können diese Tapezügel zusätzlich angelegt werden z. B. bei akuten starken Schmerzen oder langen Armen.

Mehr über die Anwendung von Basis Tape und Optionalem Tape lesen Sie auf den folgenden Seiten.

Tip on procedure

First affix the base tapes (as described) and wait for 1–2 days. The optional tape tails are then additionally affixed according to how the symptoms then present.

In this way, the taping can be tailor-made for the symptoms. Once the tape has been worn for about 1 week, the last tail should not be affixed when the new tape is applied. If several tape tails have been affixed, please omit the last tail week by week until no tape is needed anymore. Depending on the symptoms, the taping can be applied up to 4–6 times (with the tape changed once a week).

The tape length should be gauged as shown in the pictures.

Base tape*:* this tape tail should always be applied.

Optional tape: these tape tails can be applied additionally if required, e.g. for acute severe pain or on long arms.

You can read more about using the base tape and optional tape on the following pages.

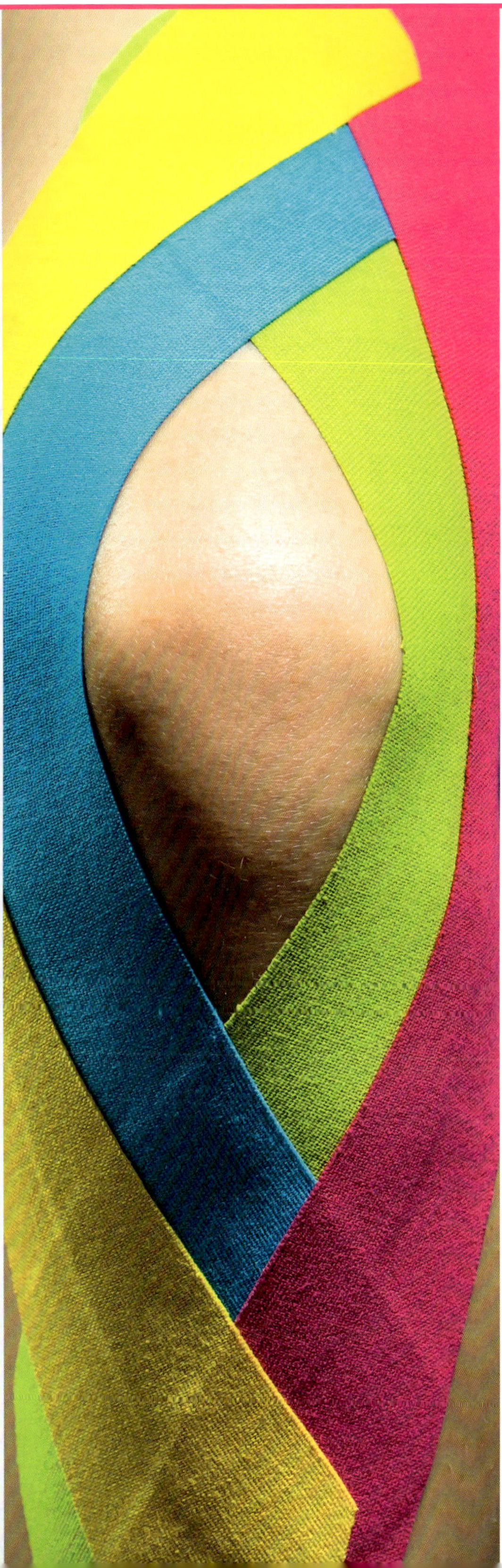

Basis Tape
Base tape

Dieses Tape bildet immer die Grundlage einer Tapeanlage.

Es sollte immer aufgeklebt werden.

This tape always forms the basis for taping.

It should always be affixed.

Optionales Tape
Optional tape

Diese Tapes können zur Verbesserung der Wirkung geklebt werden.

Sie können aber nach einer Woche Tragezeit, nach dem Tapewechsel auch mal weggelassen werden.

Der Anwender entscheidet je nach Schmerzzustand über die Notwendigkeit dieser Tapes.

These tapes can be affixed to improve the effect.

However, after being worn for one week they can also be omitted when the tape is changed.

The user decides on the need for these tapes, depending on the level of pain.

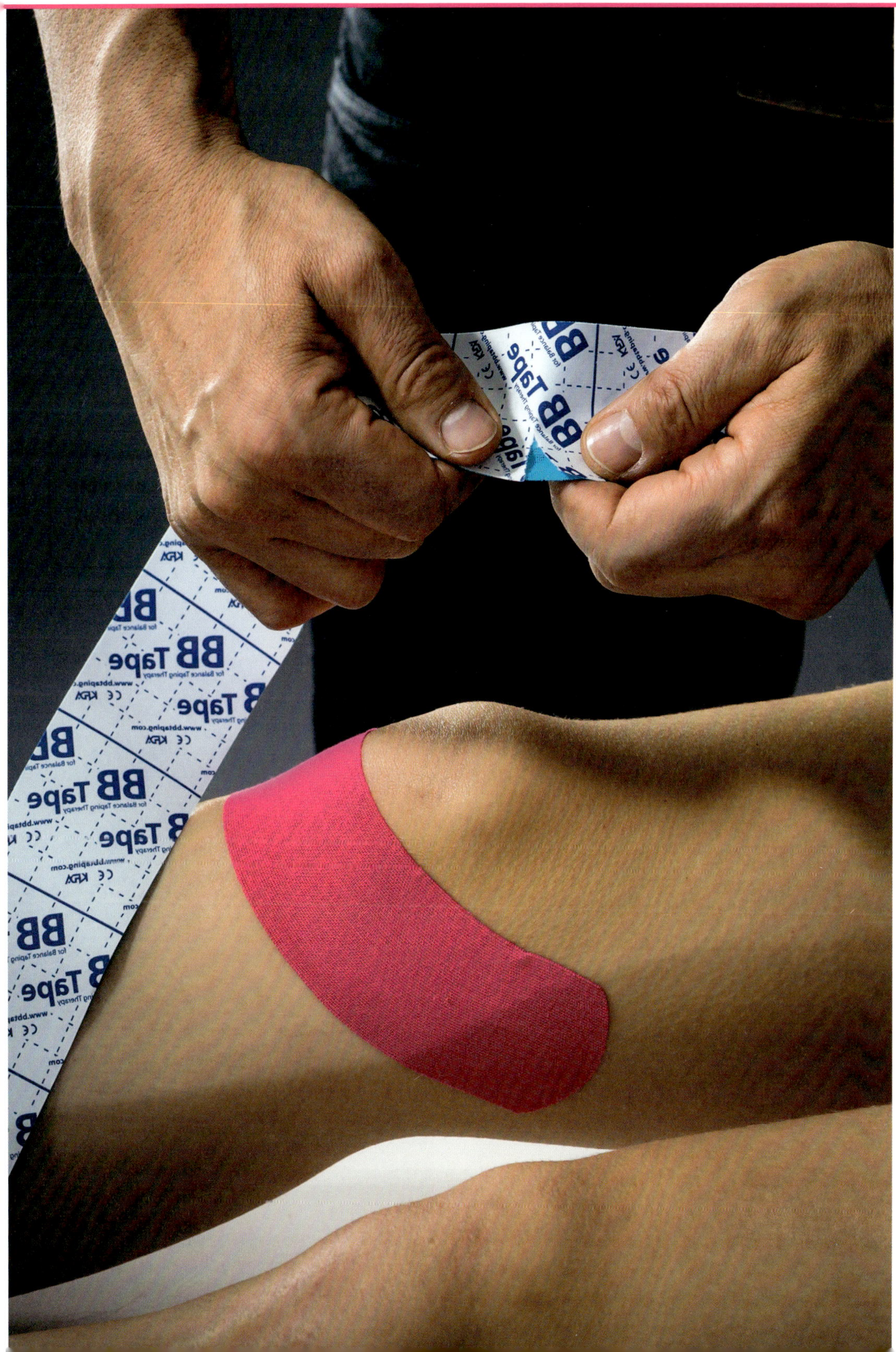
BB Tape

Vordehnen der Muskel
Pre-stretching the muscles

Dehnen ist wichtig

Wenn der Muskel durch das Tape angetriggert und der Stoffwechsel erhöht wird, dann sollte ein Tape in der Muskeltechnik angelegt werden.

Dazu müssen immer erst die betroffenen Muskeln so weit wie möglich vorgedehnt werden. Das Tape wird dann „ohne" Zug aufgeklebt.

So erreicht man den maximalen Hautabhebeffekt, wenn sich der Patient wieder in die natürliche Ausgangsstellung begibt und sich die Muskeln verkürzen.

Stretching is important

If the muscle is to be triggered and the metabolism increased by the tape, a tape should be positioned using the muscle technique.

To do so, the affected muscles must always be pre-stretched as far as possible. The tape is then affixed "without" stretch.

In this way, the maximum skin-lifting effect is obtained when the patient returns to the natural starting position and the muscles shorten.

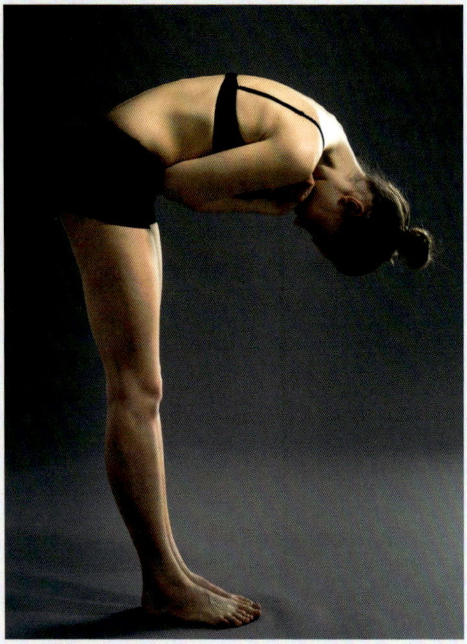

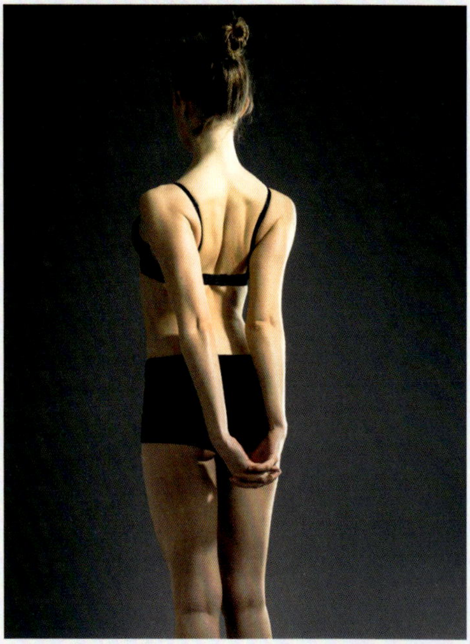

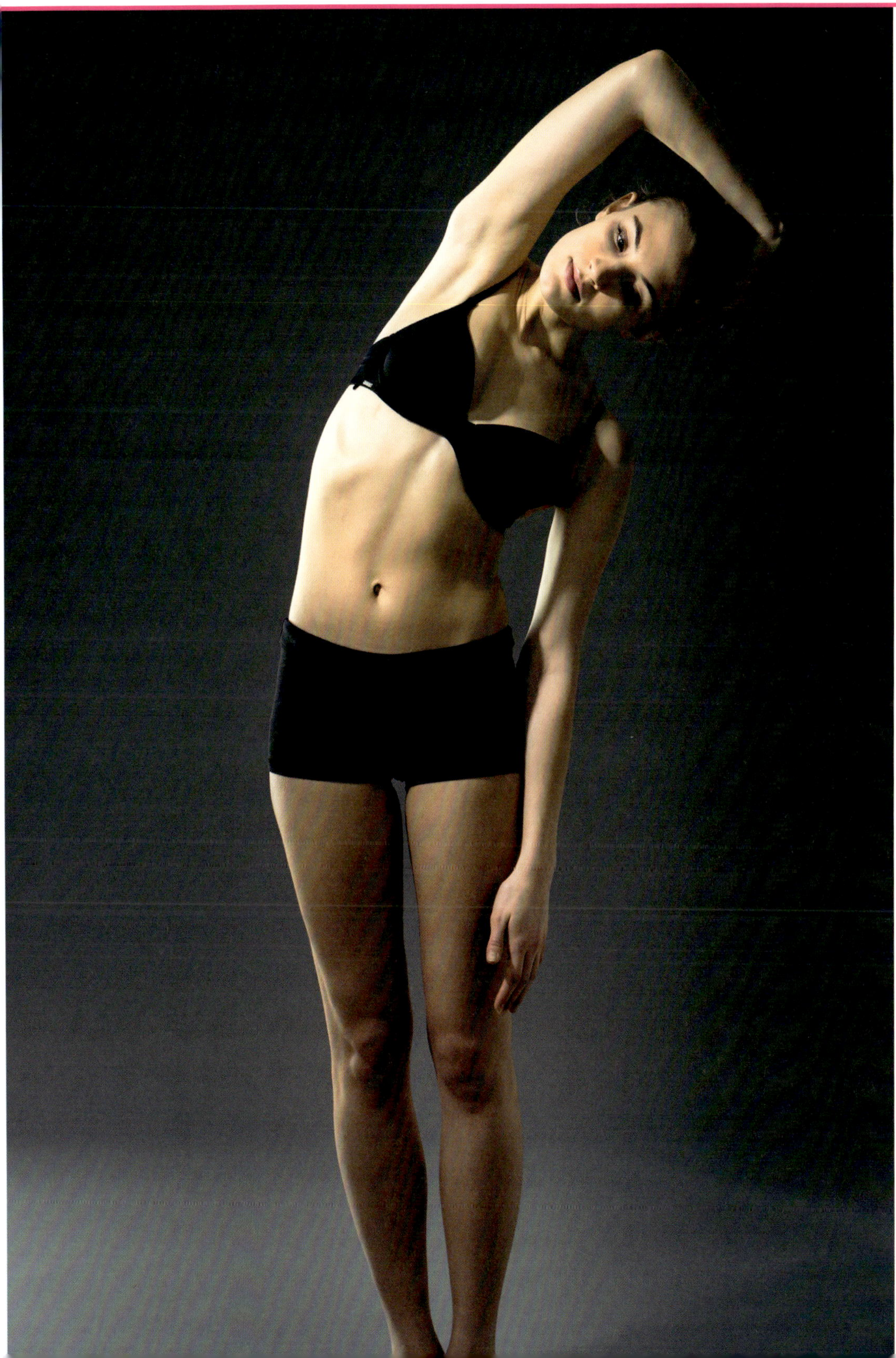

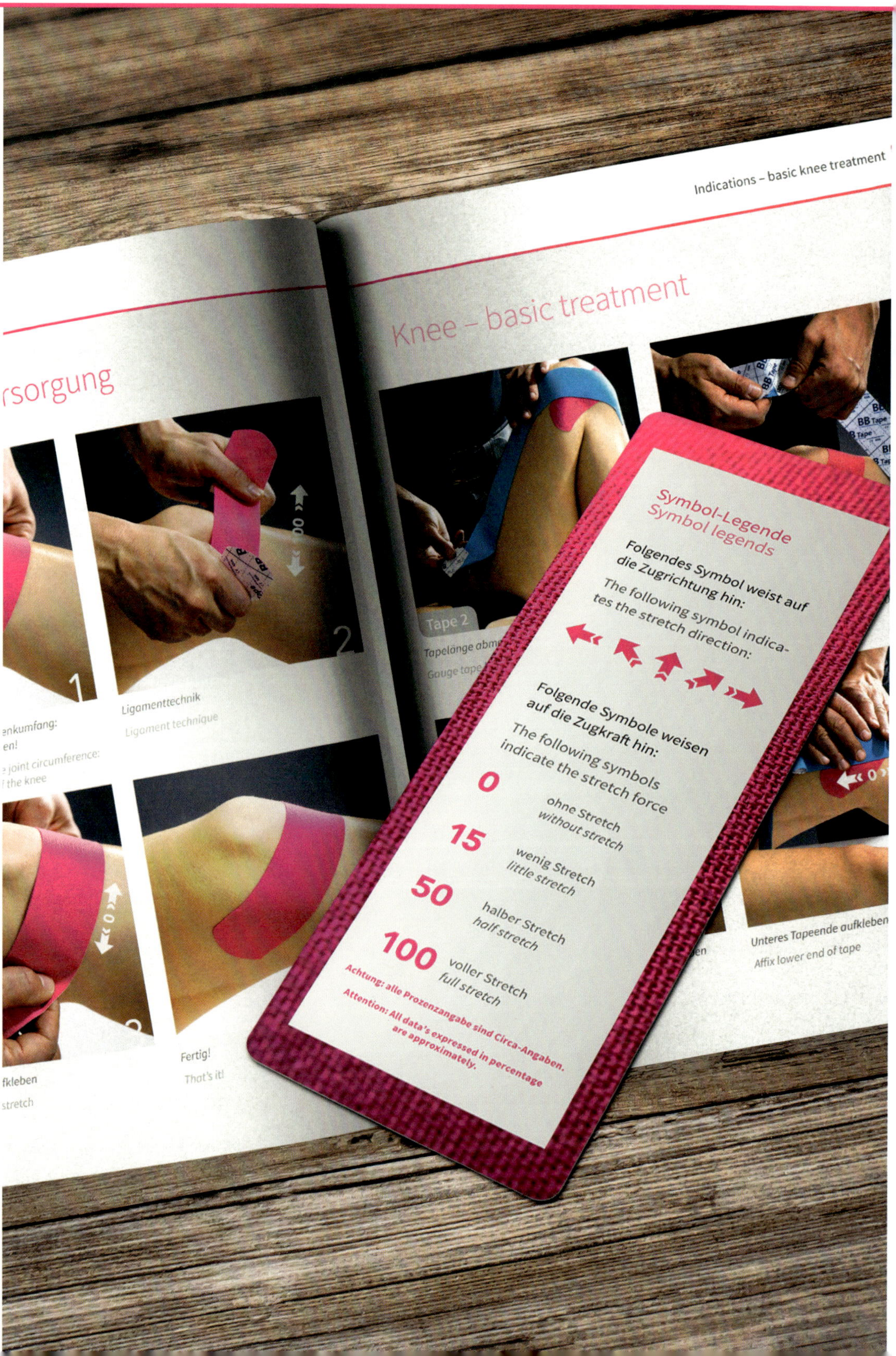
Indications – basic knee treatment
Knee – basic treatment
rsorgung
Ligamenttechnik
Ligament technique
Tape 2
Fertig!
That's it!
Unteres Tapeende aufkleben
Affix lower end of tape
Symbol-Legende
Symbol legends
Folgendes Symbol weist auf die Zugrichtung hin:
The following symbol indicates the stretch direction:
Folgende Symbole weisen auf die Zugkraft hin:
The following symbols indicate the stretch force
0 ohne Stretch without stretch
15 wenig Stretch little stretch
50 halber Stretch half stretch
100 voller Stretch full stretch
Achtung: alle Prozenzangabe sind Circa-Angaben.
Attention: All data's expressed in percentage are approximately.

Symbole-Legende
Symbol legends

Folgendes Symbol weist auf die Zugrichtung hin

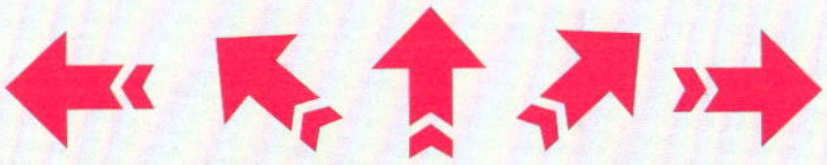

Folgende Symbole weisen auf die Zugkraft hin

0 (ohne Stretch)

15 (wenig Stretch)

50 (halber Stretch)

100 (voller Stretch)

Achtung: Alle Prozenzangabe sind Circa-Angaben.

- **Mit 15 % oder 30 % ist gemeint: leichten Stretch auf das Tape geben.**
- **Bei 50 %: Tape erst bis zum Maximum ausdehnen, dann zur Hälfte zurücklassen und aufkleben.**
- **Bei 100 % ist der maximale Stretch gemeint, welches das Tape zulässt.**

The following symbol indicates the stretch direction

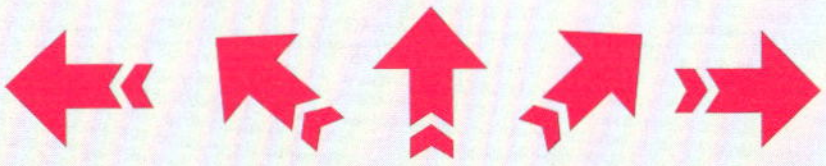

The following symbols indicate the stretch force

0 (without stretch)

15 (little stretch)

50 (half stretch)

100 (full stretch)

Attention: All data's expressed in percentage are approximately.

- **15% or 30% means: affix the tape with little stretch.**
- **50% means: First pull the tape with maximum stretch, then go back 50% and apply the tape.**
- **100% means: Use the whole stretch of the tape according to how elastic the tape is.**

Tennisarm Basis Tape
Tennis elbow base tape

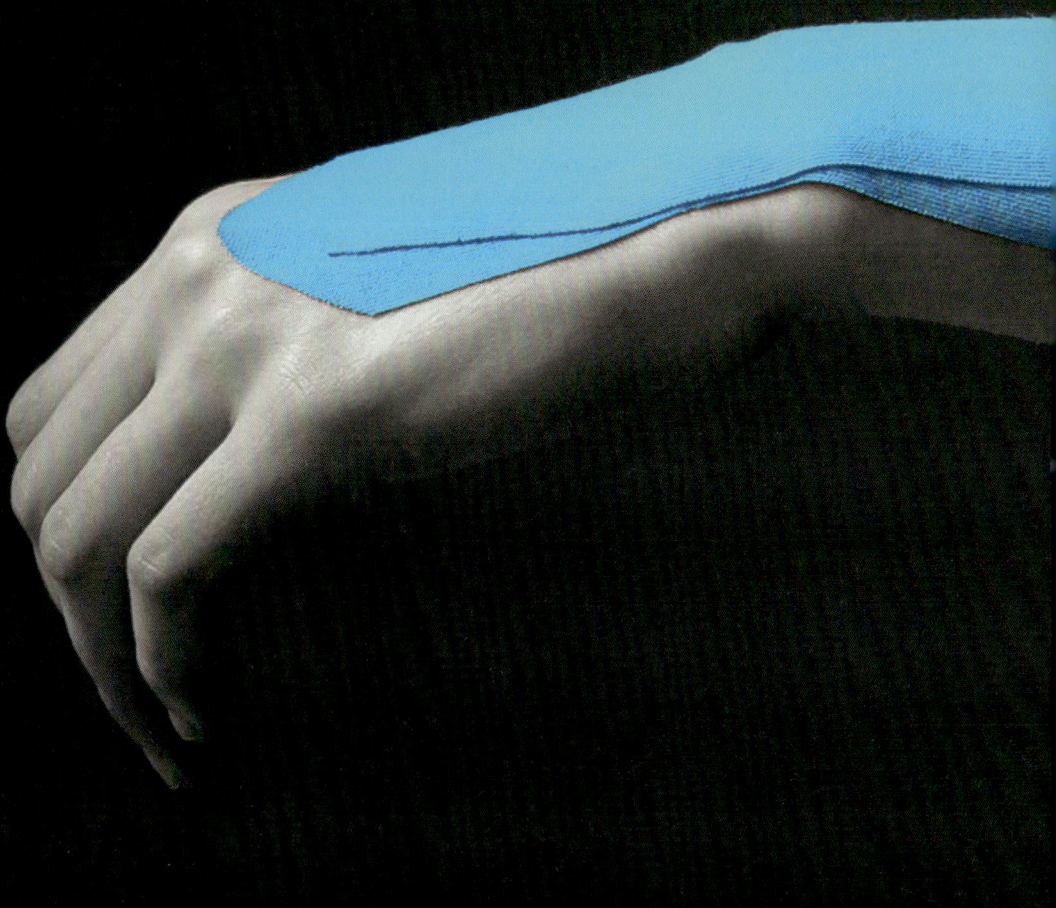

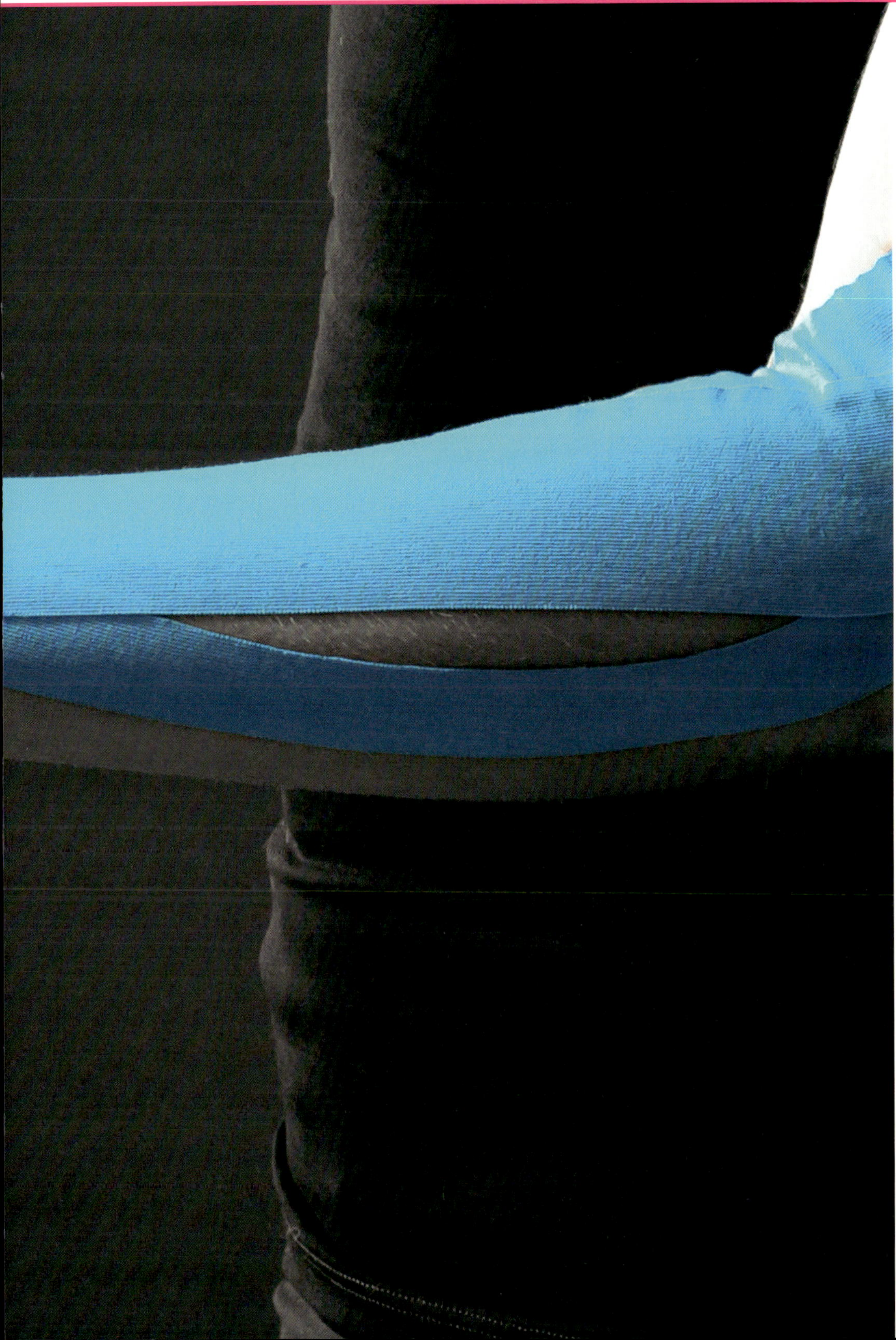

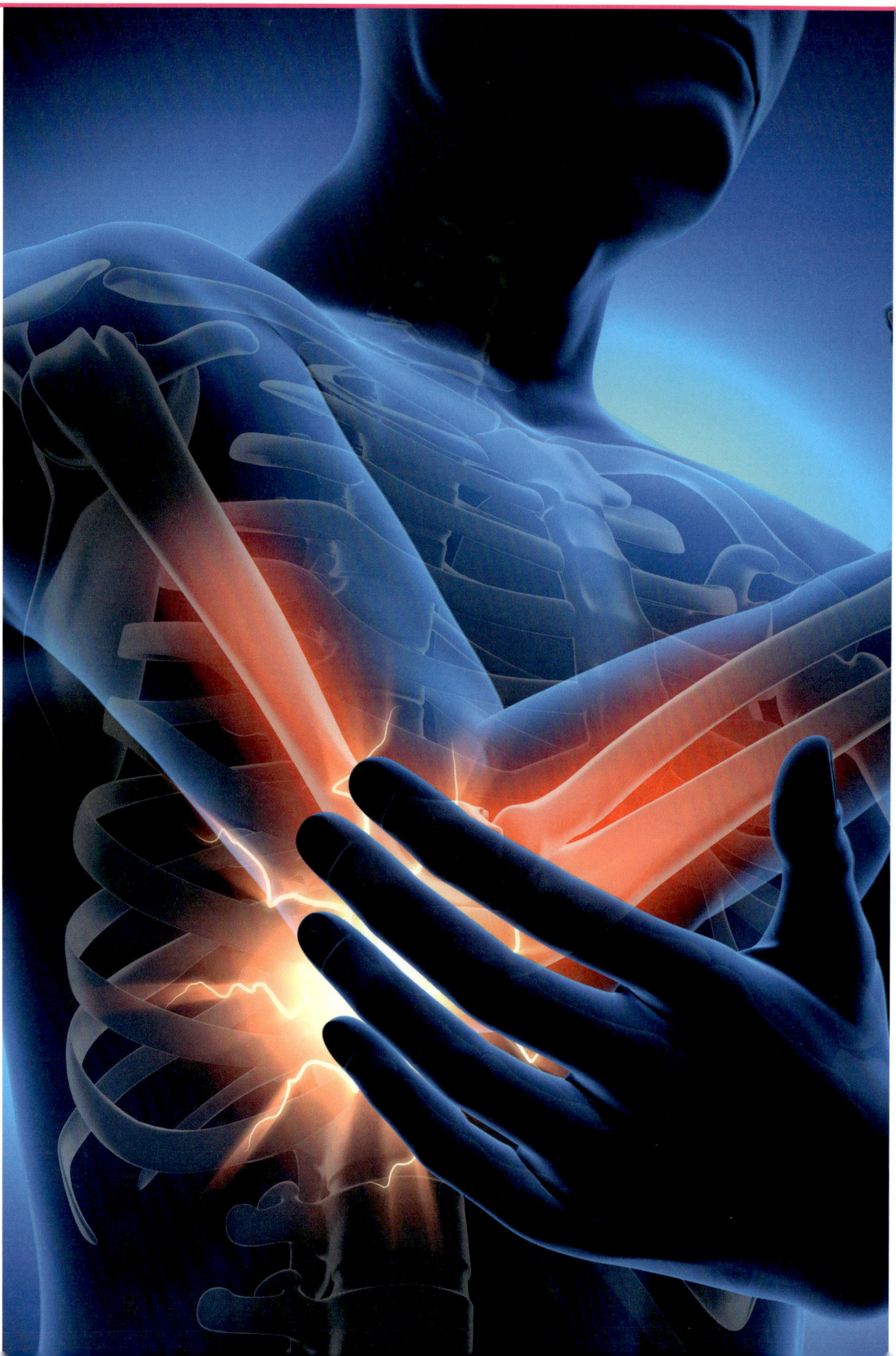

Tennisarm
Tennis elbow

Hinweise

Das Tape wird angelegt bei:

- Schmerzen an den Handstreckern, unter anderem beim sogenannten Tennsiarm

Das gleiche Tape kann angelegt werden bei:

- Sehnenscheidenentzündungen
- Überlastungssyndrome in der Muskulatur
- Zur Entlastung des Handgelenkes

Advice

The tape is applied for:

- Pain in the forearm extensor muscles, including the condition called tennis elbow

The same tape can be applied for:

- Tendon sheath inflammation
- Muscle overuse syndrome
- Wrist decompression

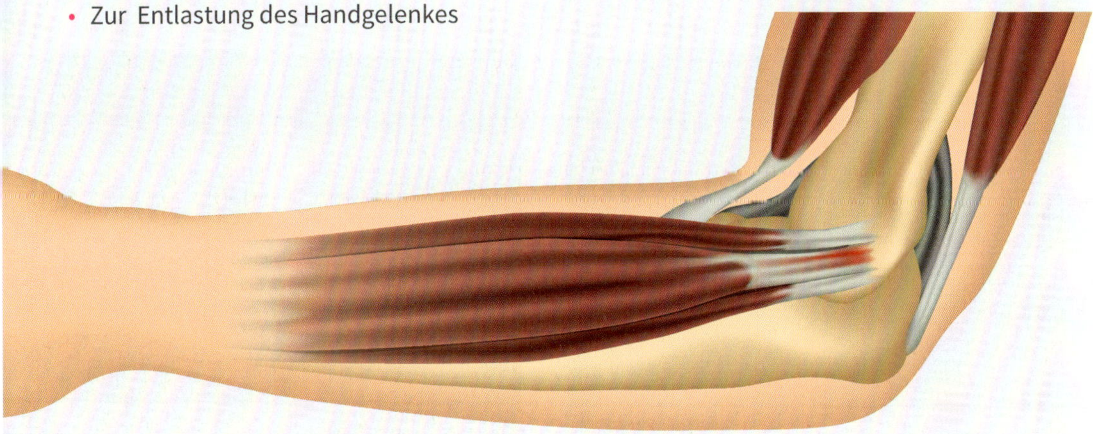

Bitte nutzen Sie die Gitterpflaster zur Wirkungsverbesserung vor jeder Anwendung. Einfach auf die Schmerzpunkte kleben

Please use the cross-tapes to improve the effect prior to each application Simply affix to the painful spots

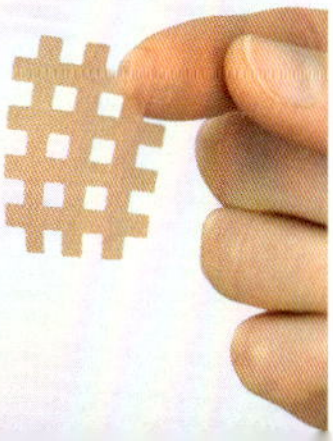

Tennisarm – Basistape

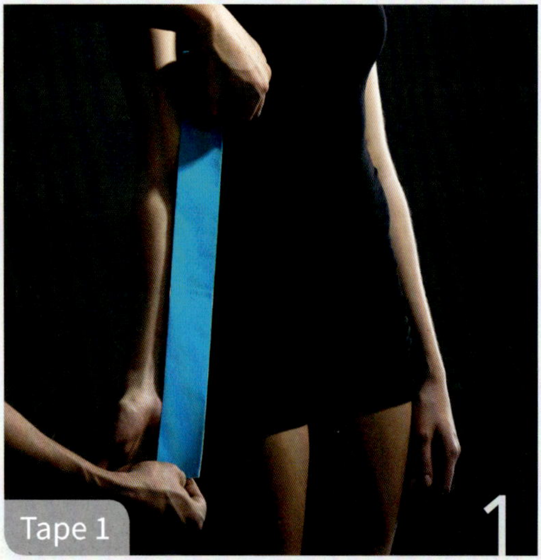

Tapelänge abmessen (Länge siehe Foto)

Gauge tape length (for length, see photo)

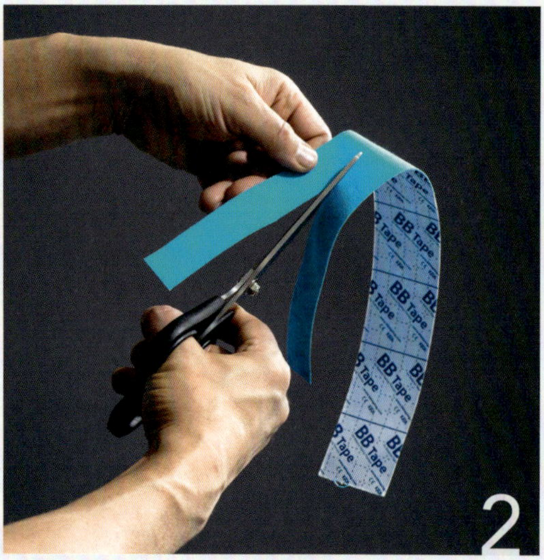

Tape bis auf 5 cm einschneiden

Cut the tape except for 5 cm

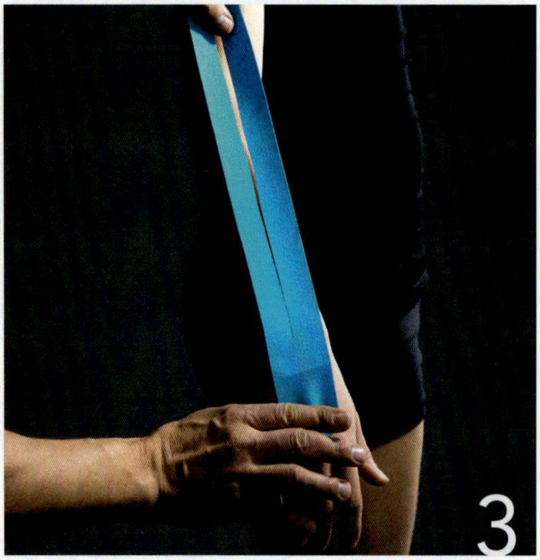

Tapebasis auf dem Handrücken aufkleben

Affix base tape to the back of the hand

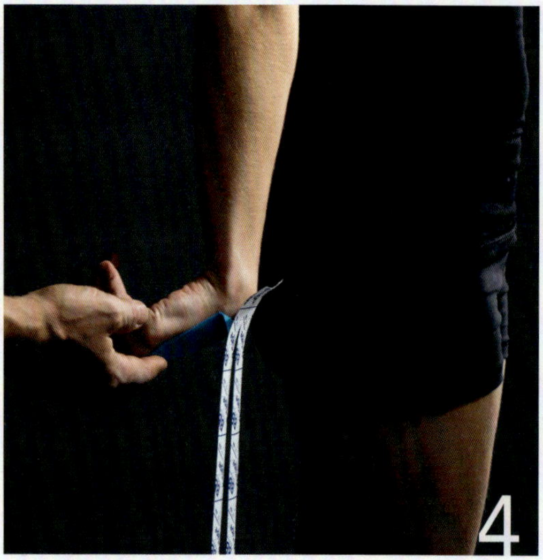

Muskeln vordehnen

Pre-stretch the muscles

Tennis elbow – base tape

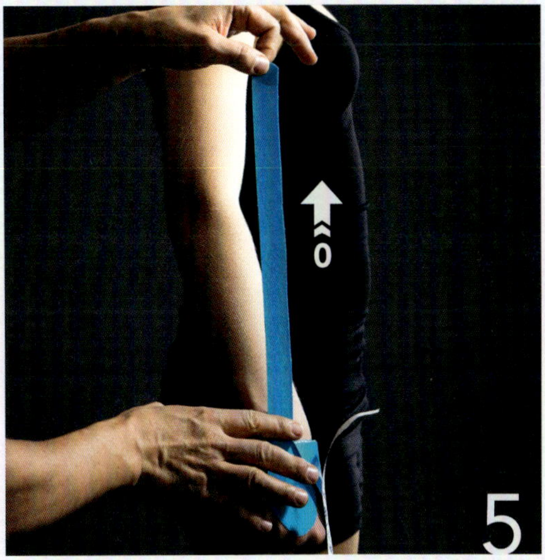

Linken Tapezügel um die Muskeln am Unterarm anlegen

Position left-hand tape tail around the forearm muscles

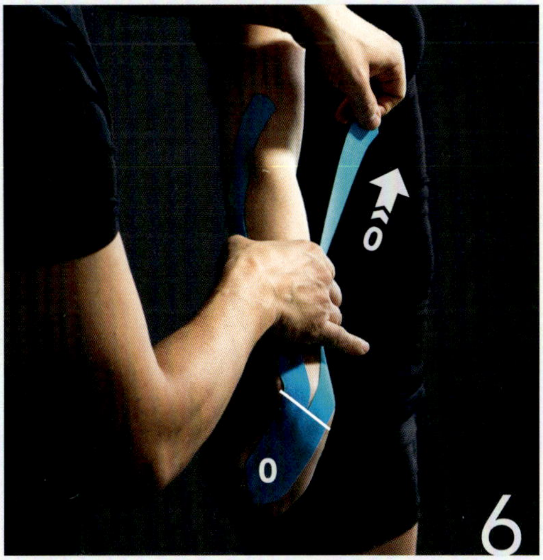

Rechten Tapezügel um die Muskeln am Unterarm anlegen

Position right-hand tape tail around the muscles on the forearm

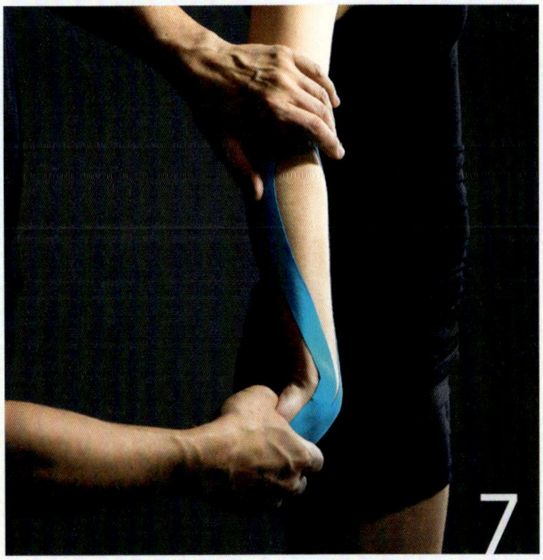

Tape anreiben

Rub down the tape

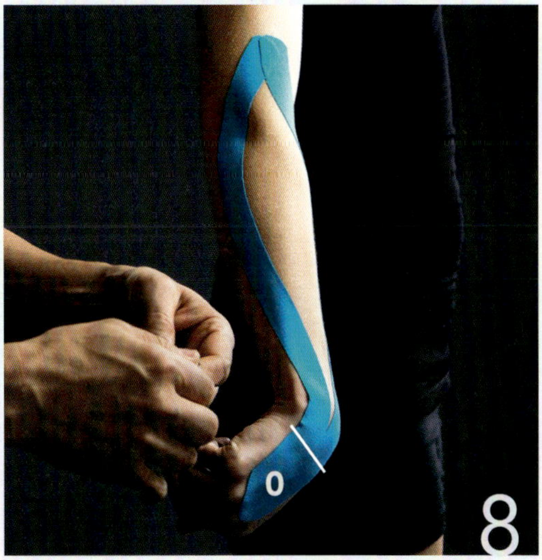

Fertig!

That's it!

Tennisarm
Tennis elbow

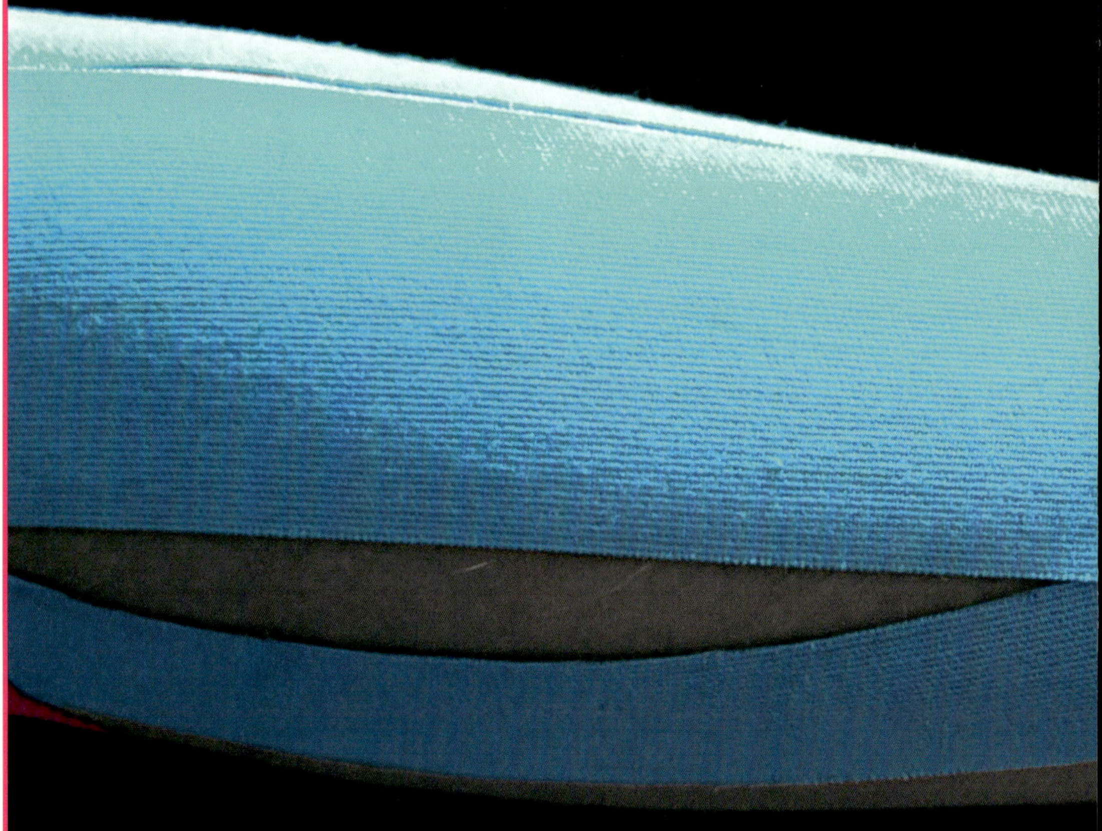

Optionale Tapes

Besonders geeignet bei starken Schmerzen

optional tapes

Ideal in case for severe pain

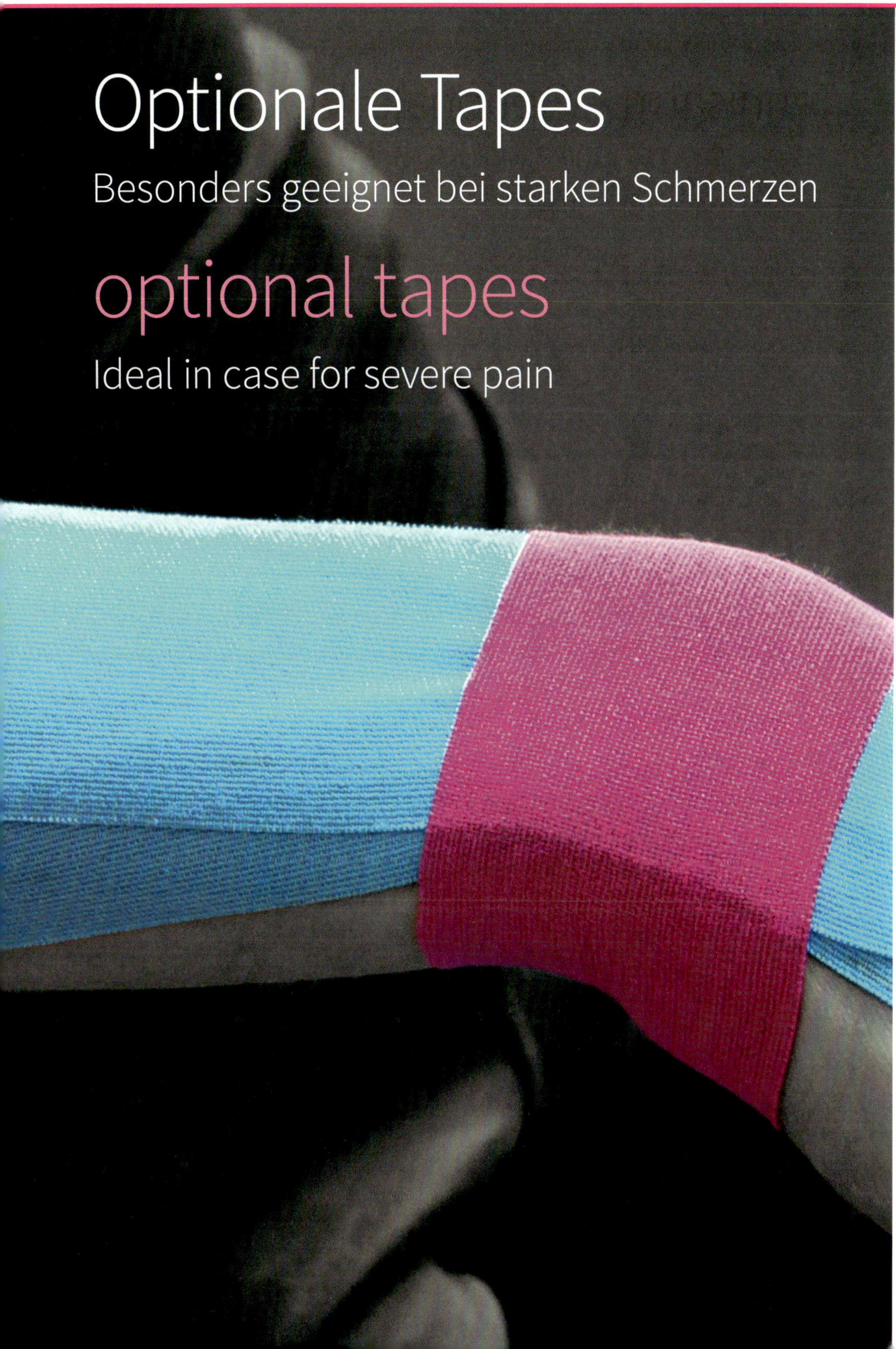

Tennisarm – Optionale Tapes

Zur lokalen Schmerzentlastung auf dem Epikondylus

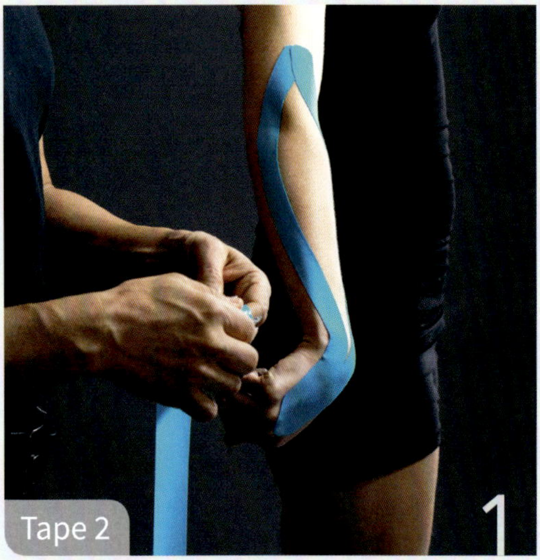

Kompaktes Tape: Auf dem Handrücken aufkleben

Compact tape: affix to the back of the hand

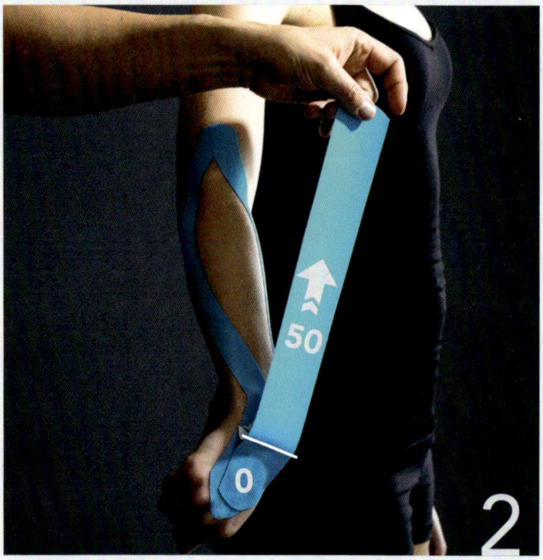

Muskel vordehnen

Pre-stretch the muscle

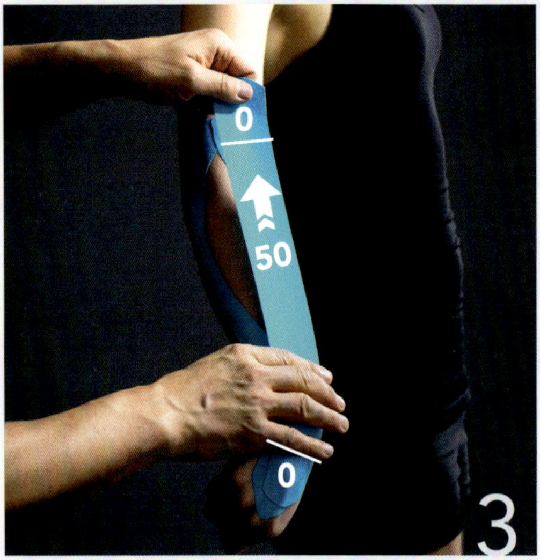

Tape mit 50 % Zug aufkleben

Affix tape with 50% stretch

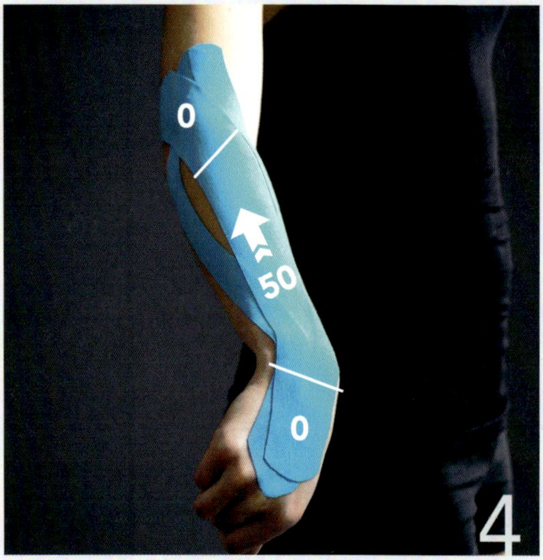

Fertig!

That's it!

Tennis elbow – optional tapes

To alleviate local pain on the epicondyle

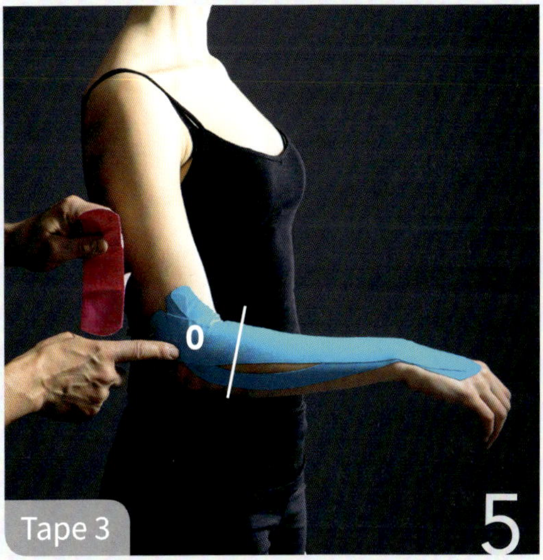

Schmerzpunkt

Painful spot

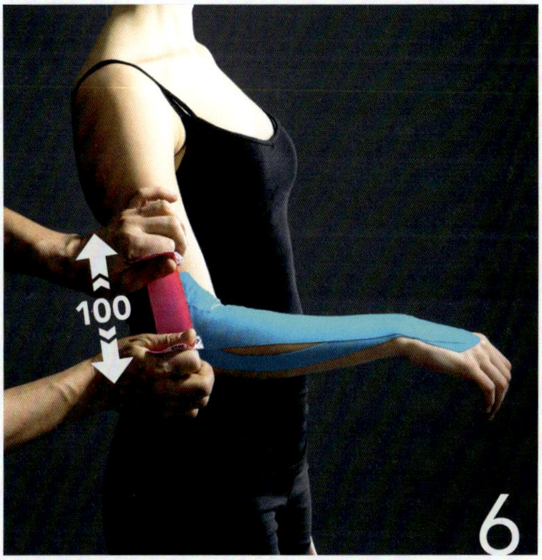

Ligamenttechnik

Ligament technique

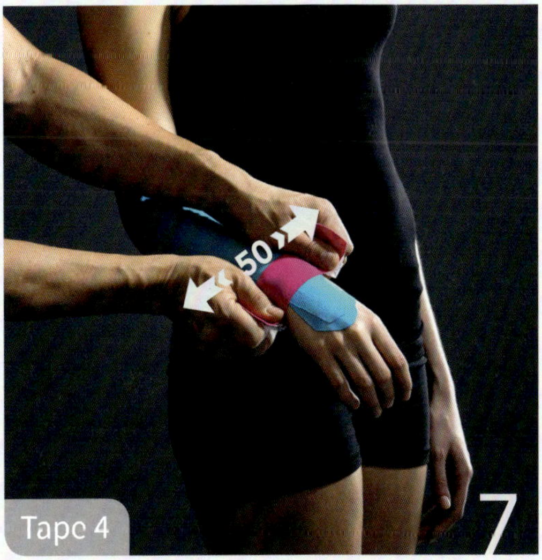

Ligamenttechnik dient zur Fixierung

Ligament technique in order to fix the tape

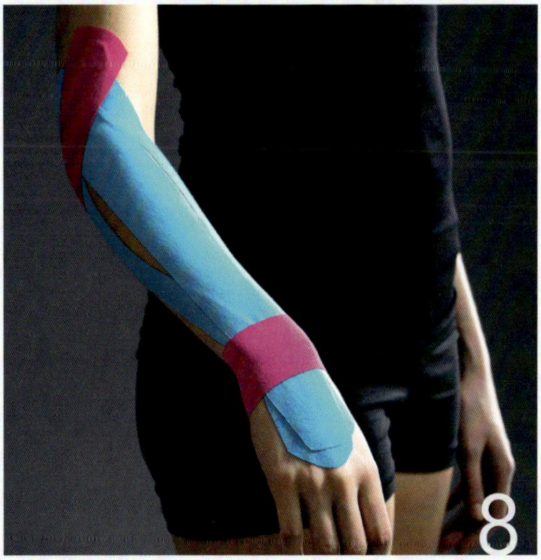

Fertig!

That's it!

Golferarm und Karpaltunnelsyndrom Basis Tape

Golfer's elbow and carpal tunnel syndrome base tape

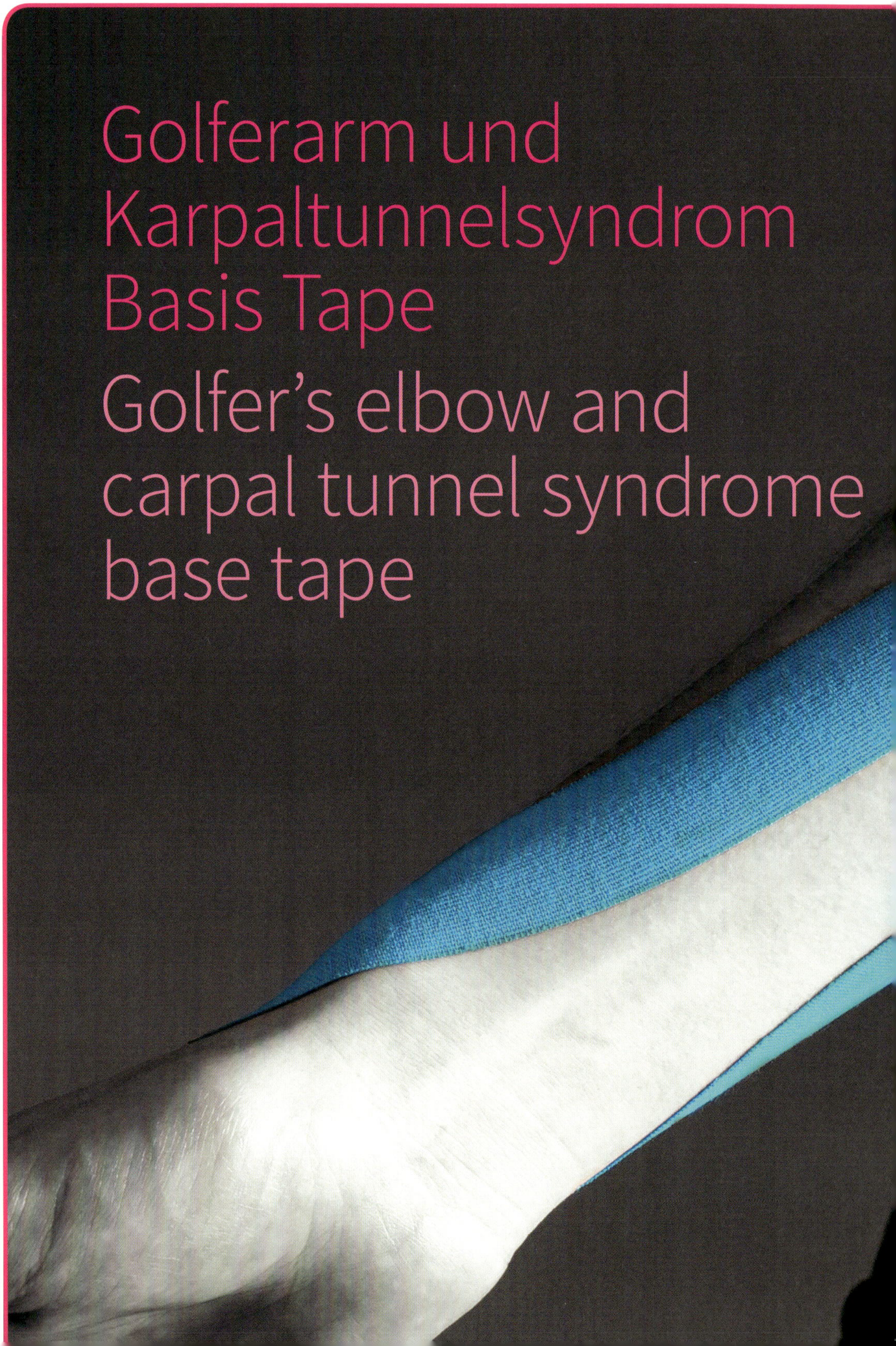

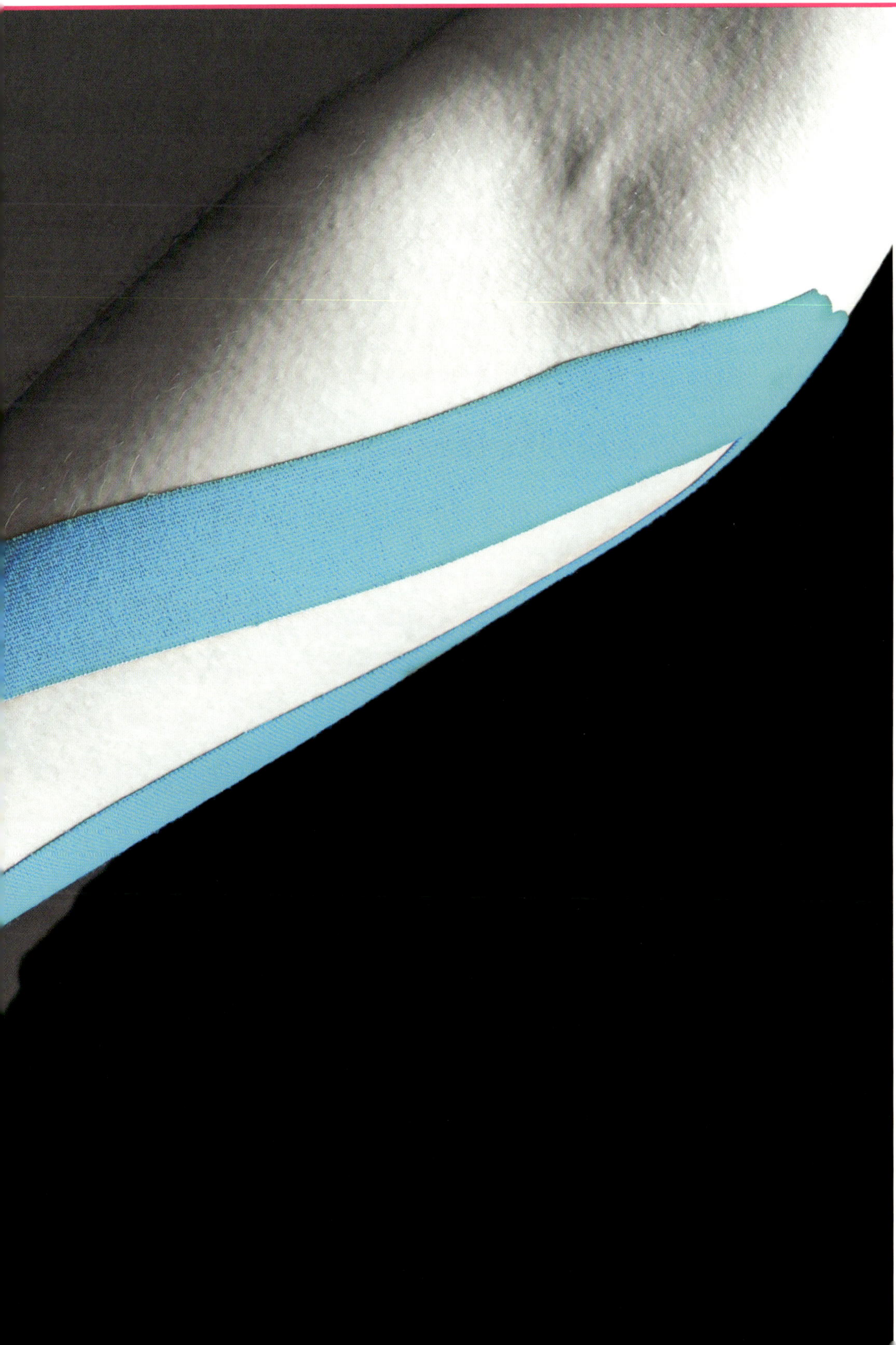

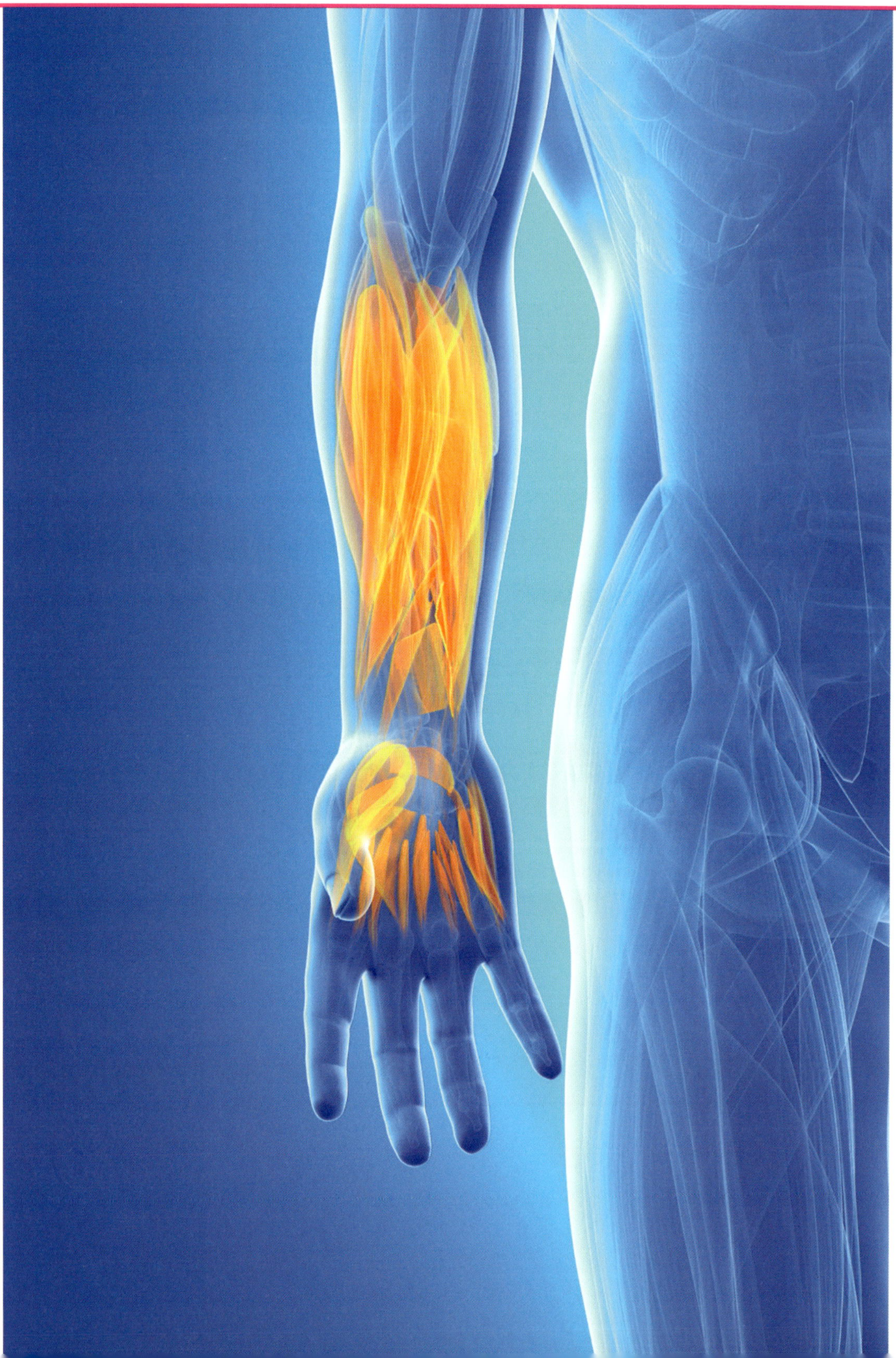

Golferarm und Karpaltunnelsyndrom
Golfer's elbow and carpal tunnel syndrome

Hinweise

Dieses Tape kann das Karpalband entlasten. Der Mittelarmnerv hat wieder Platz. Tape 3–4 mal anwenden.

Außerdem wird das Tape angelegt bei:

- Schmerzen in den Fingern
- Schmerzen im Handgelenk
- Ruheschmerzen

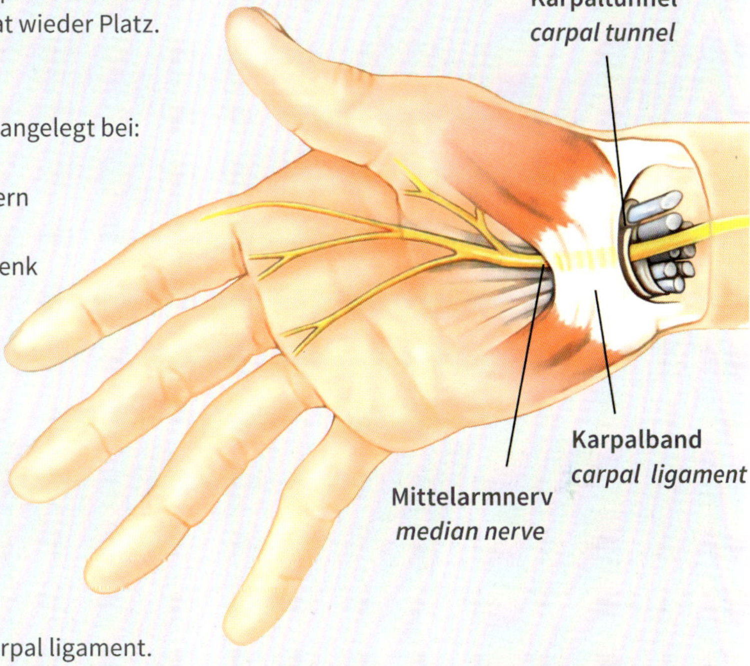

Advice

This tape can relieve the carpal ligament. The middlearm nerve has sufficient space again. Apply the tape 3-4 times.

Additional the tape will be used by:

- Pain in fingers
- Pain in wrist
- Rest pain

Bitte nutzen Sie die Gitterpflaster zur Wirkungsverbesserung vor jeder Anwendung. Einfach auf die Schmerzpunkte kleben

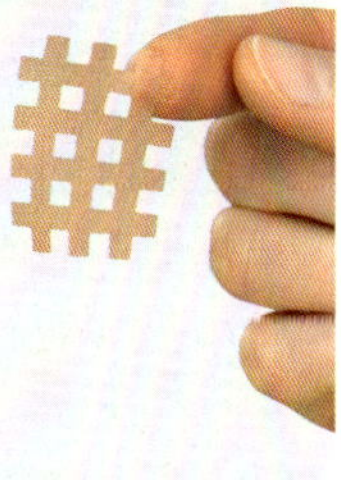

Please use the cross-tapes to improve the effect prior to each application Simply affix to the painful spots

Golferarm und Karpaltunnelsyndrom – Basis Tape

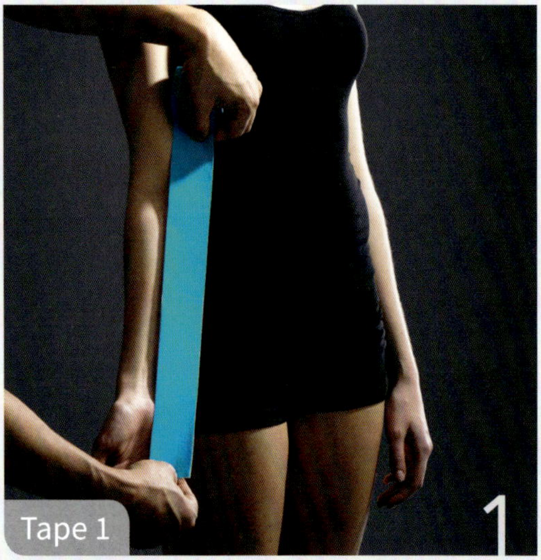

Tapelänge abmessen

Gauge tape length

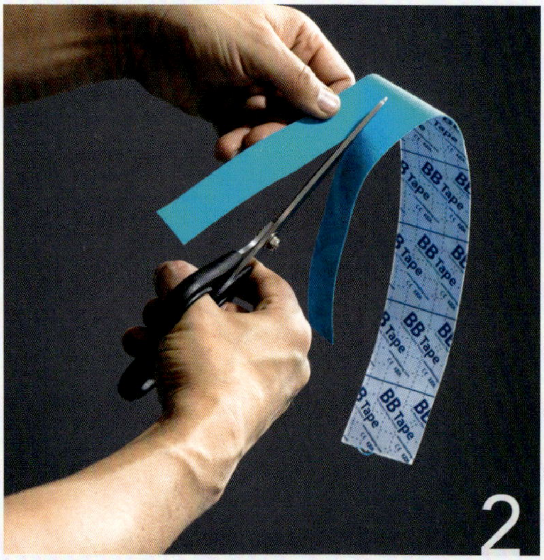

Tape bis auf 5 cm der Länge nach halbieren

Halve tape lengthways, leaving 5 cm at the end

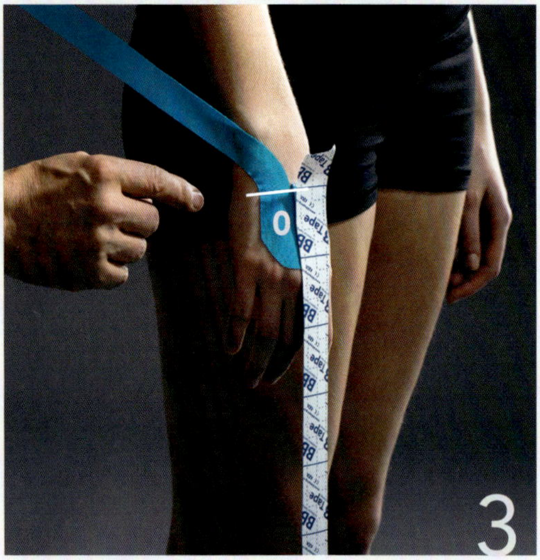

Tapebasis auf dem Handrücken bis über das Handgelenk aufkleben

Affix base tape to the back of the hand up to the wrist

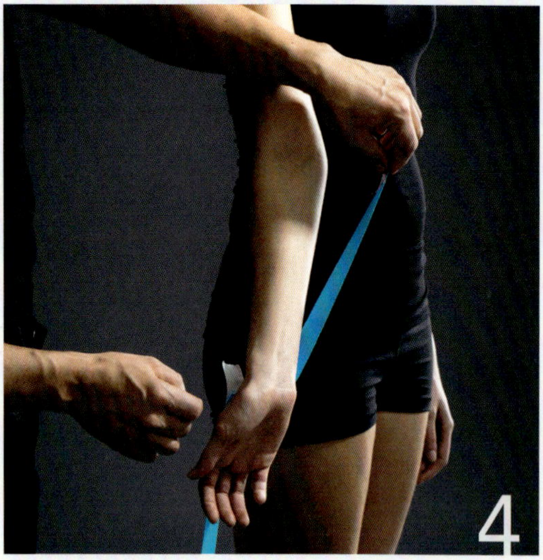

Muskeln vordehnen

Pre-stretch the muscles

Golfer's elbow and carpal tunnel syndrome – base tape

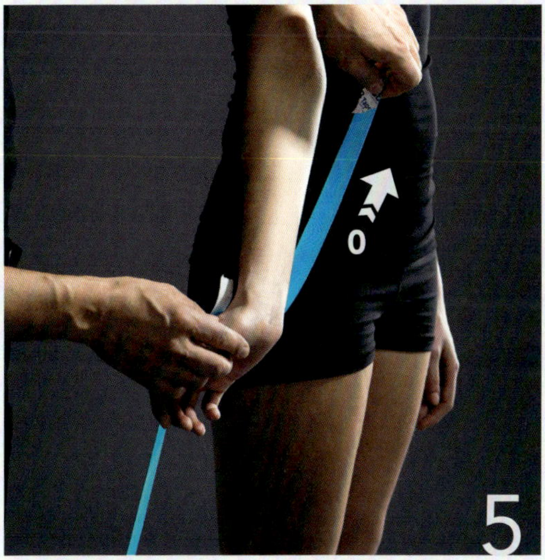

Tapezügel innen um die Muskeln anlegen

Position tape tails around the inside of the muscles

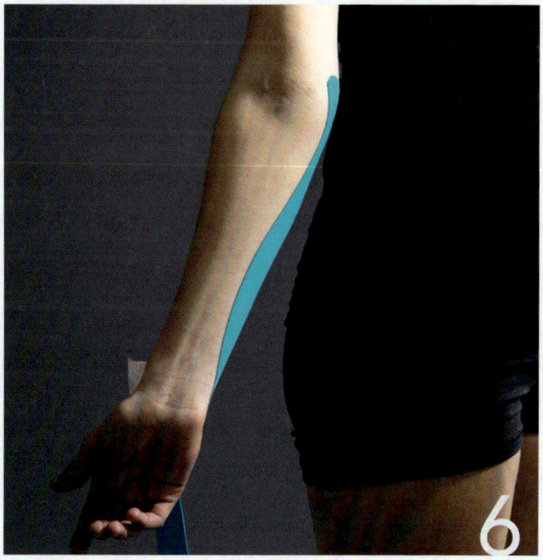

Tape bis über den Epikondylus laufen lassen

Run the tape just over the epicondyle

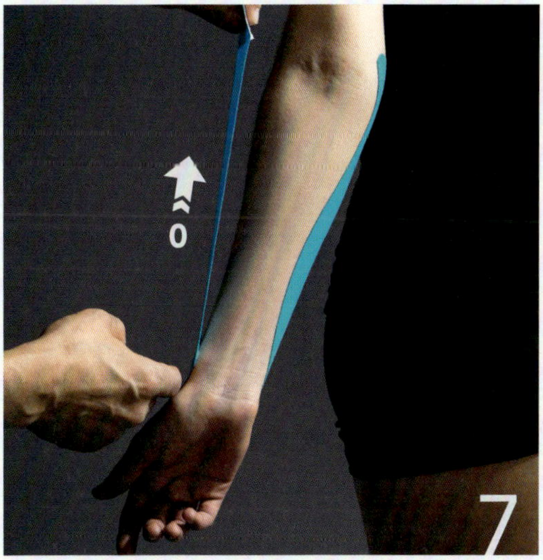

Tapezügel außen um die Muskeln anlegen

Position tape tails around the outside of the muscles

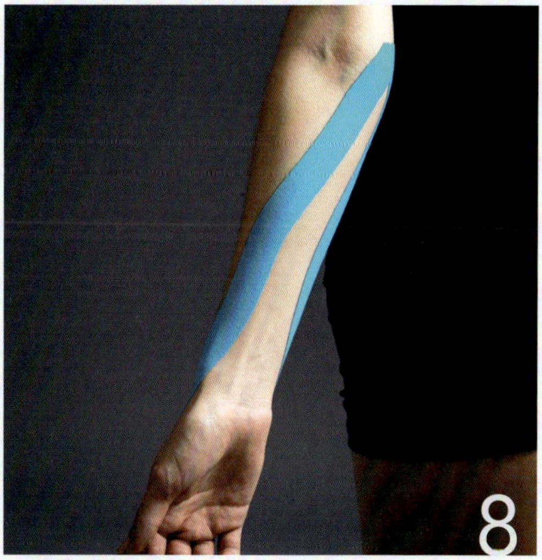

Tape anreiben

Rub down the tape

Golferarm und Karpaltunnelsyndrom Optionale Tapes

Besonders geeignet bei starken Schmerzen

Golfer's elbow and carpal tunnel syndrome optional tapes

Ideal in case of severe pain

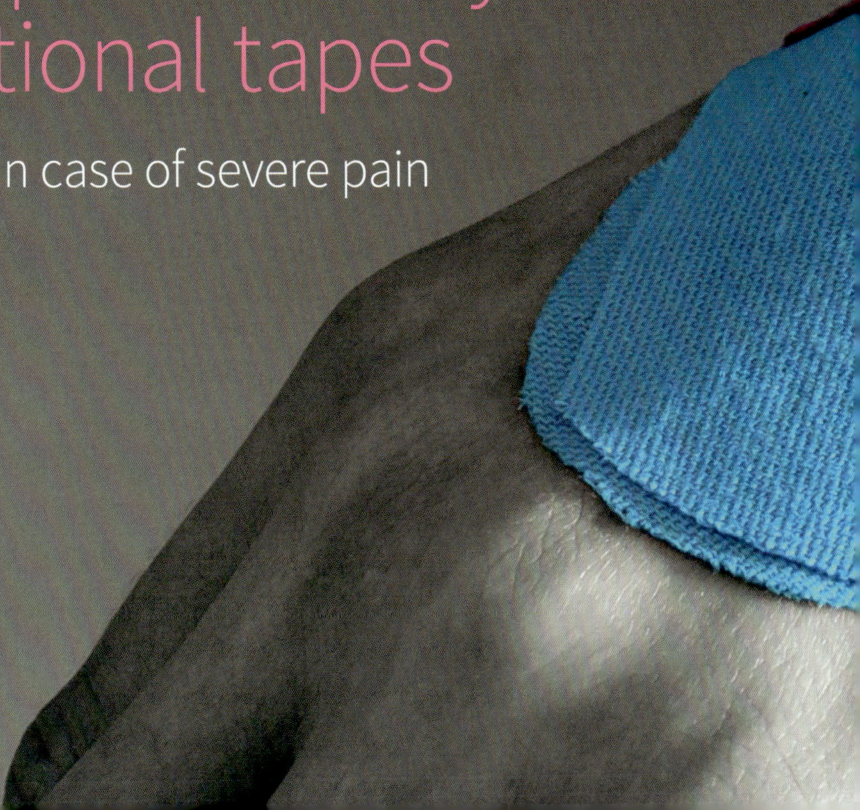

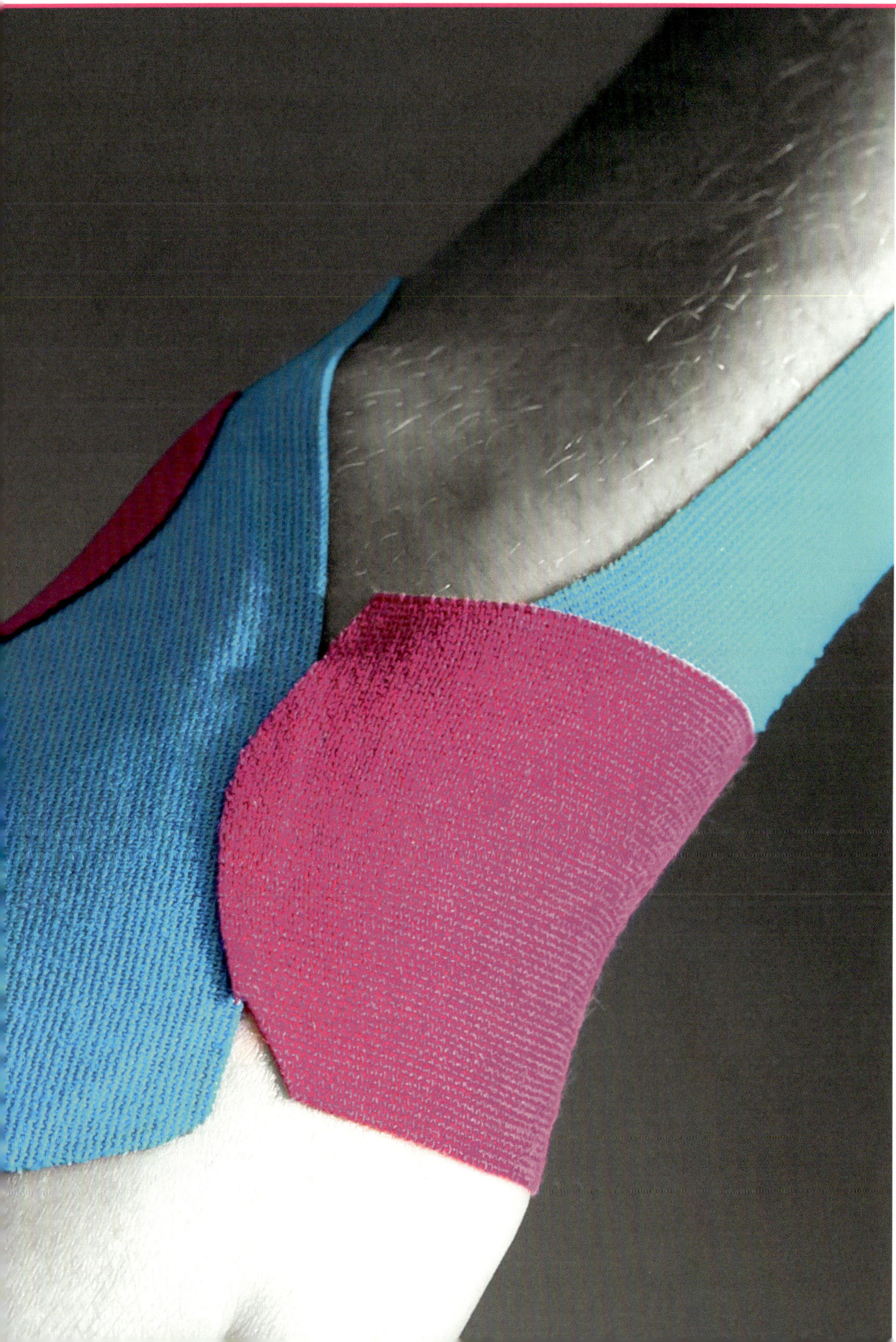

Golferarm und Karpaltunnelsyndrom

Dieser Tape dient zur zusätzlichen Schmerzentlastung.

Tipp: Nur bei starken, akuten Schmerzen in der 1. Woche aufkleben.

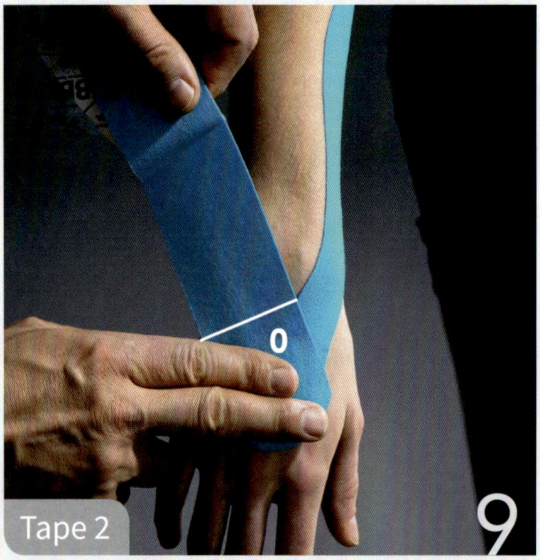

Kompakter Tape: Auf dem Handrücken aufkleben

Compact tape: affix to the back of the hand

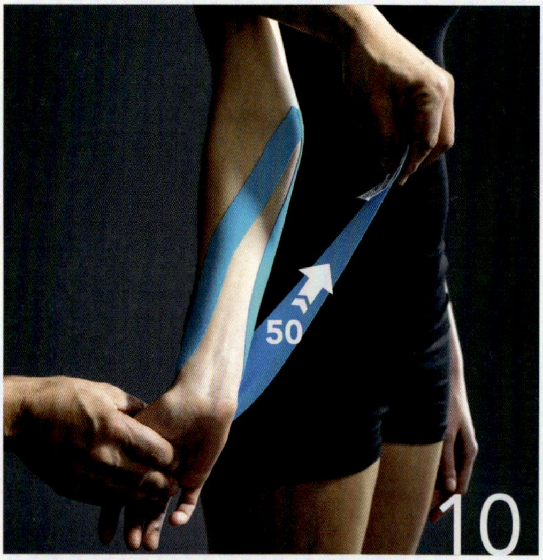

Muskeln vordehnen

Pre-stretch the muscles

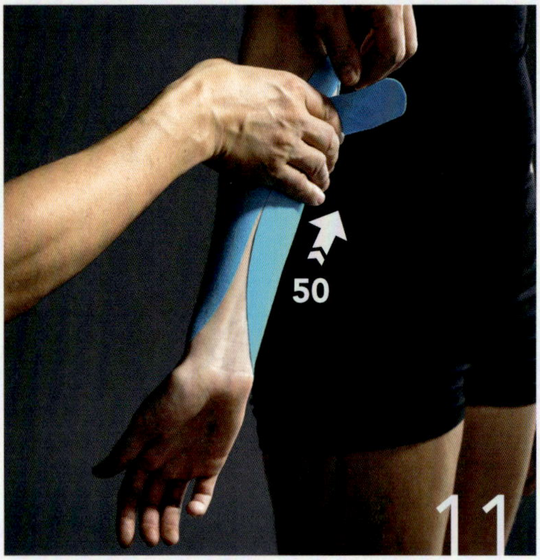

Tape aufkleben

Affix tape

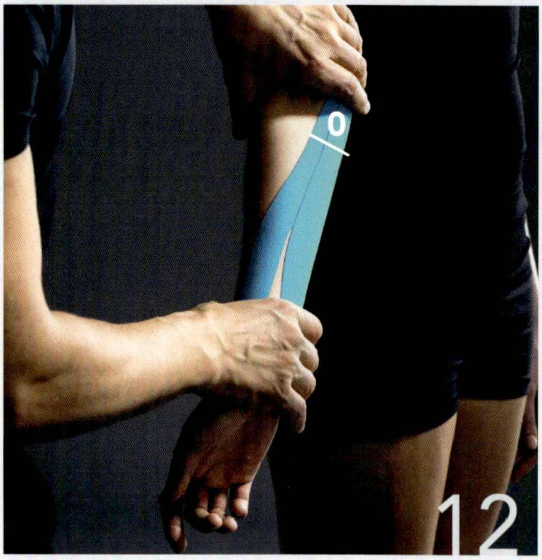

Fertig!

That's it!

Golfer's elbow and carpal tunnel syndrome

This tape provides additional pain relief.

Tip: affix in the 1st week only for severe acute pain.

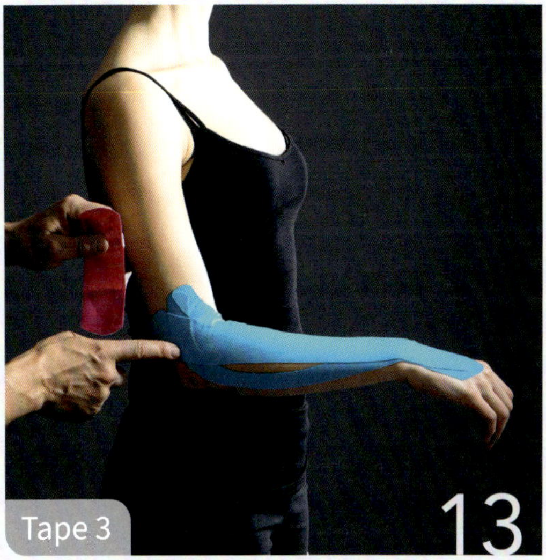

Ligamenttechnik

Ligament technique

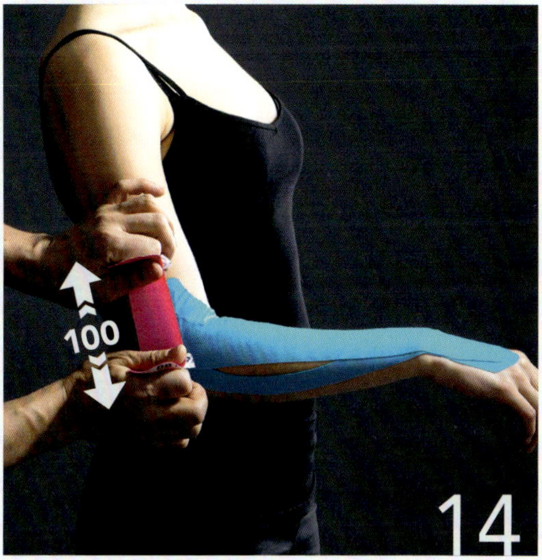

Ligamenttechnik

Ligament technique

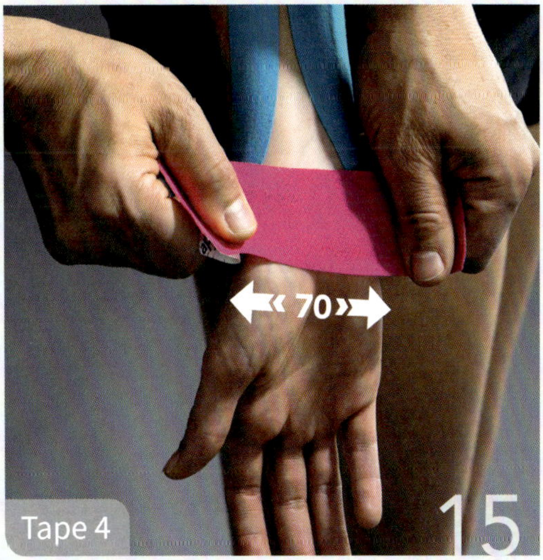

Ligamenttechnik

Ligament technique

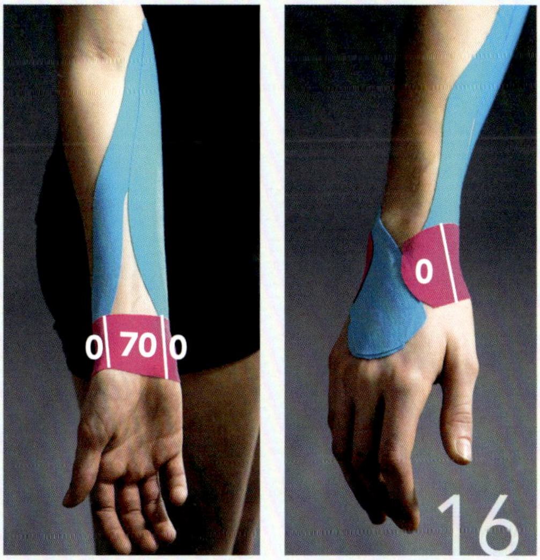

Fertig!

That's it!

Knie – Basisversorgung
Knee – basic treatment

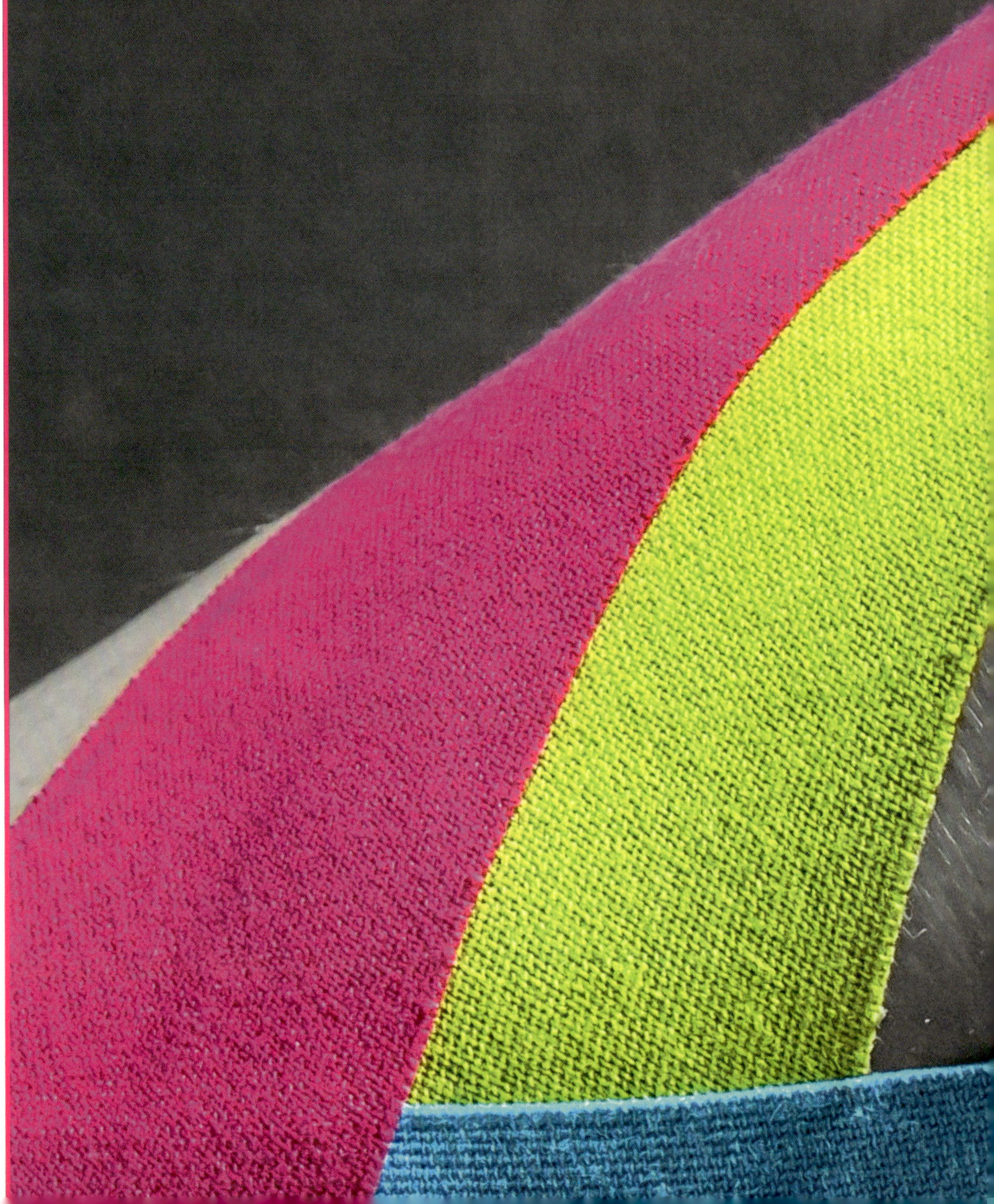

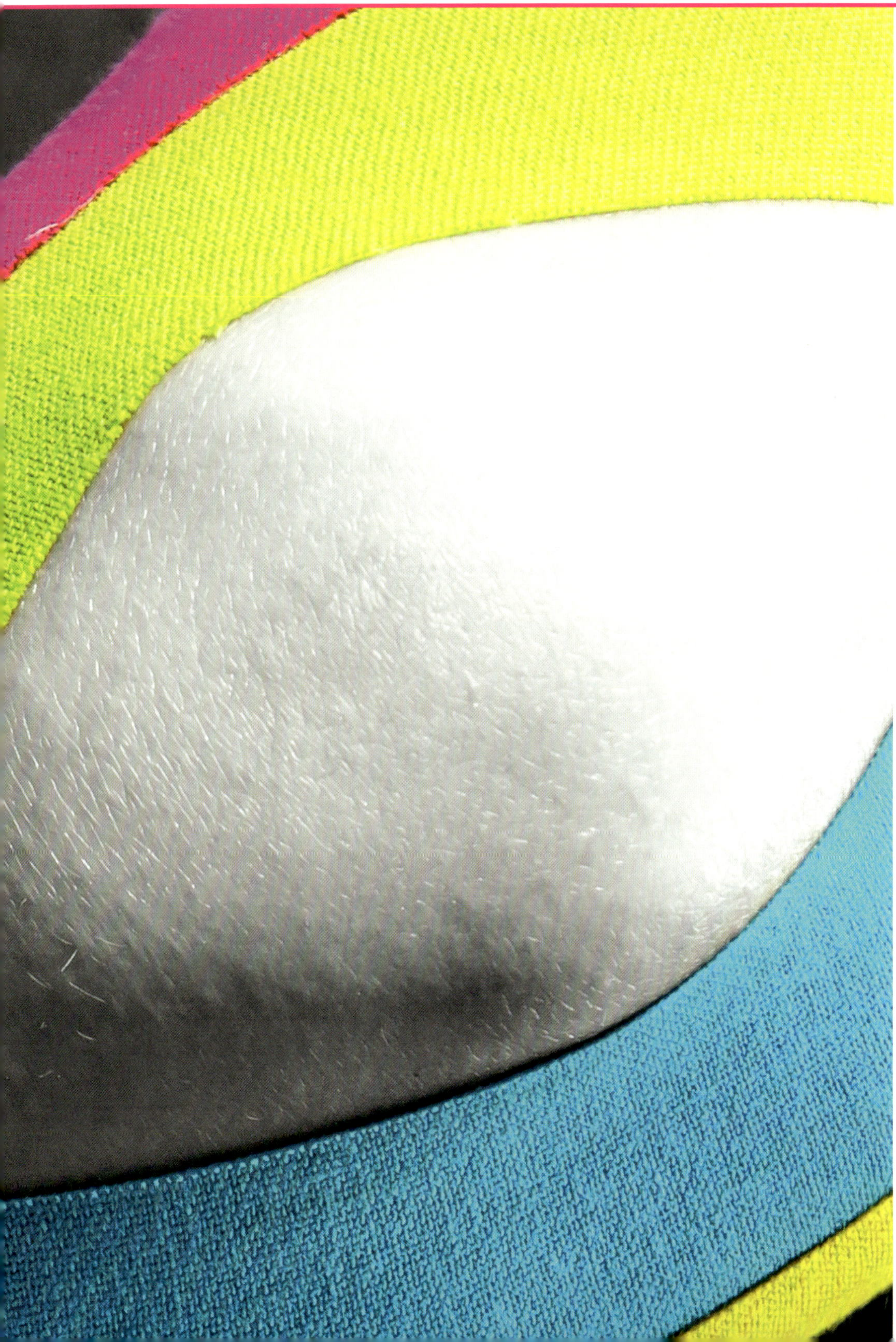

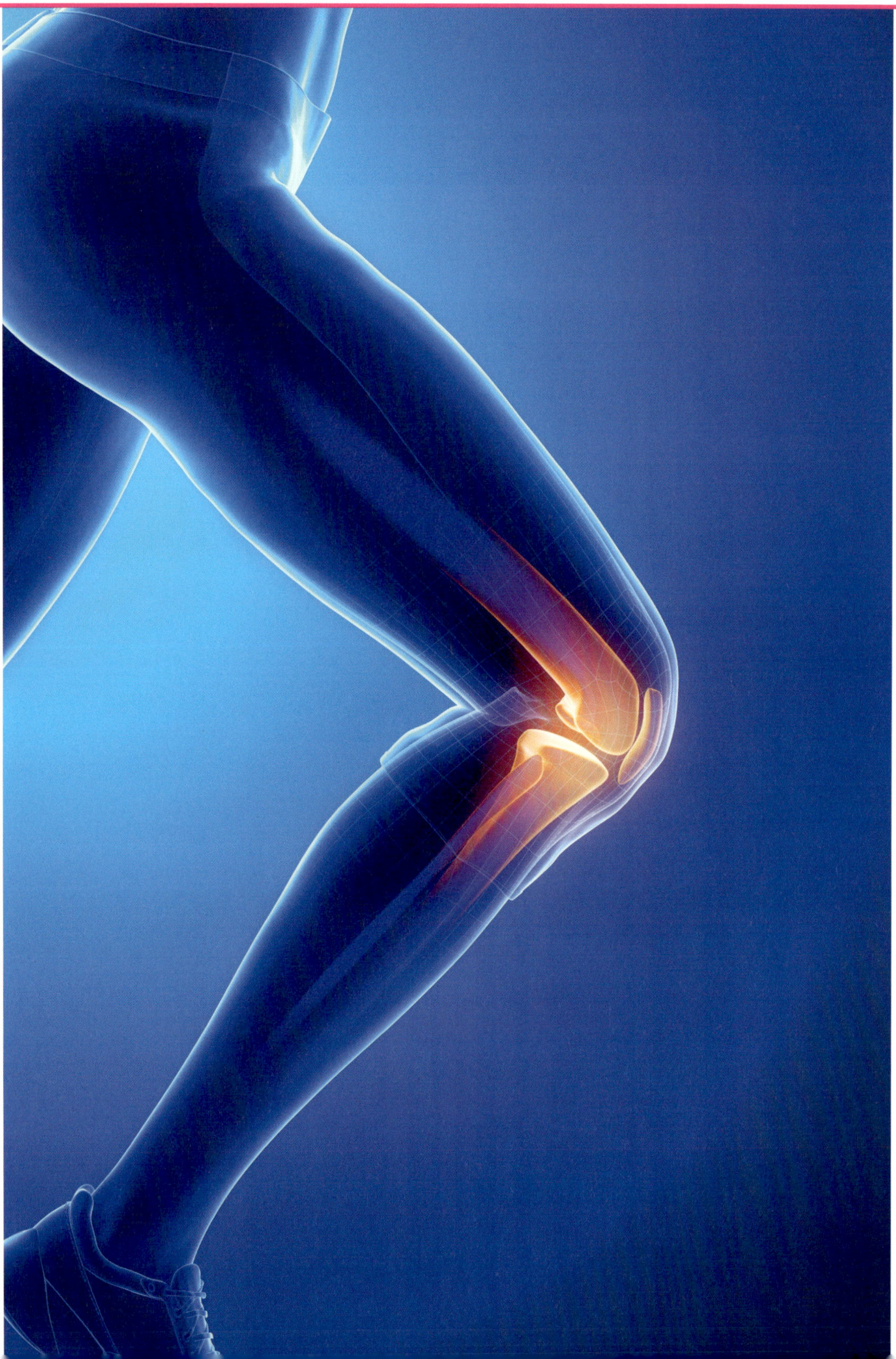

Das Knie
The knee

Hinweise

Das Tape wird angelegt bei:

- allen Beschwerden am Knie
- nach Verletzungen
- nach Knie TEP
- Innen- und/oder Außenband-beschwerden
- Belastungsbeschwerden
- Meniskusbeschwerden

Advice

The tape is applied for:

- all knee discomfort
- following injuries
- following total knee replacement
- medial and/or lateral collateral ligament discomfort
- weight-bearing discomfort
- meniscus discomfort

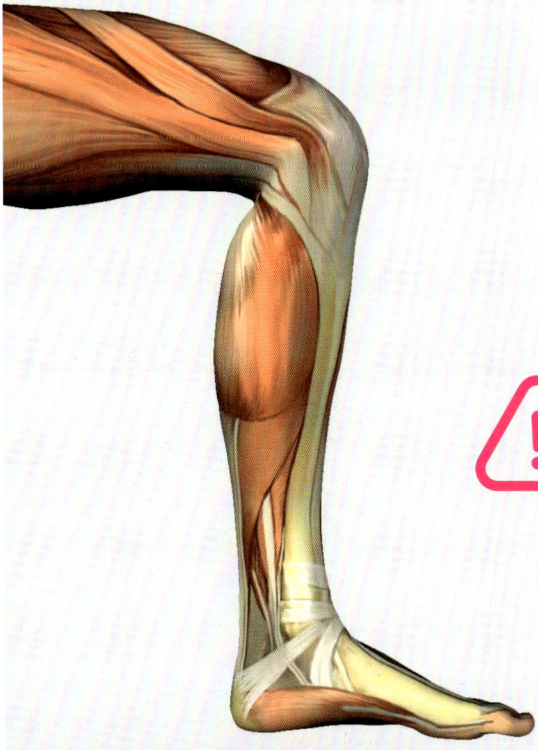

Bitte nutzen Sie die Gitterpflaster zur Wirkungsverbesserung vor jeder Anwendung. Einfach auf die Schmerzpunkte kleben

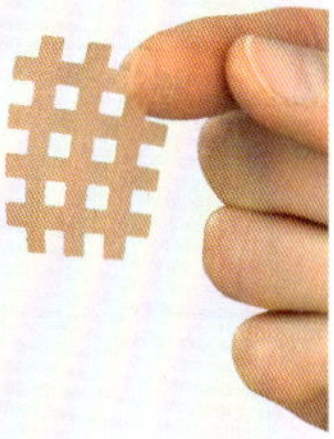

Please use the cross-tapes to improve the effect prior to each application Simply affix to the painful spots

Knie – Basisversorgung

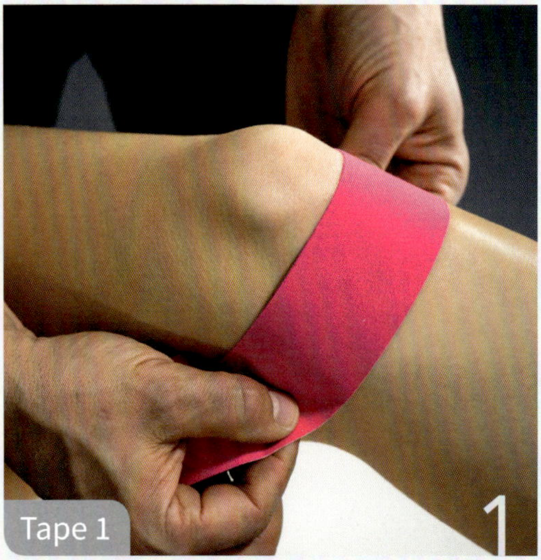

Tapelänge ist der halbe Kniegelenkumfang: Tape nicht in die Kniekehle kleben!

The tape length is half the knee joint circumference: do not affix tape to the back of the knee!

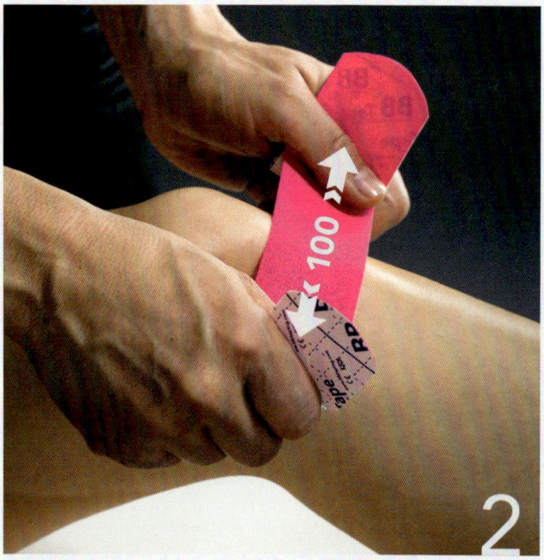

Ligamenttechnik

Ligament technique

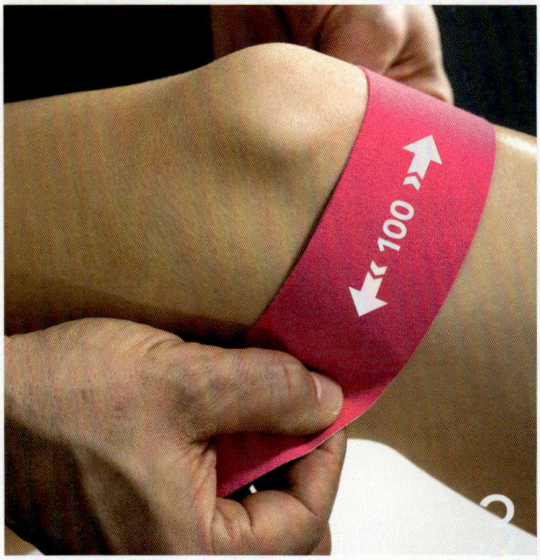

Enden ohne Zug aufkleben

Affix ends without stretch

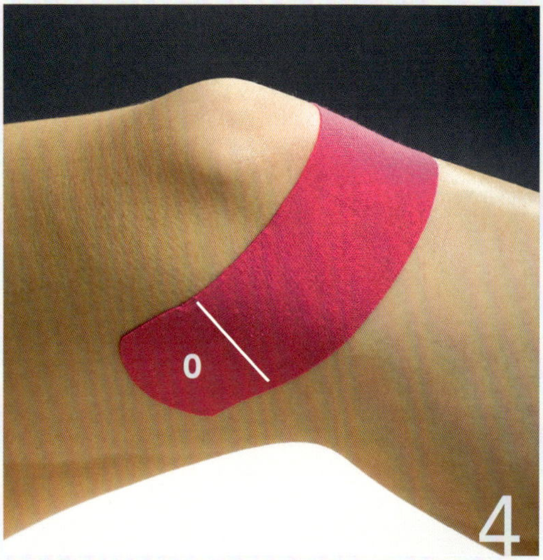

Fertig!

That's it!

Knee – basic treatment

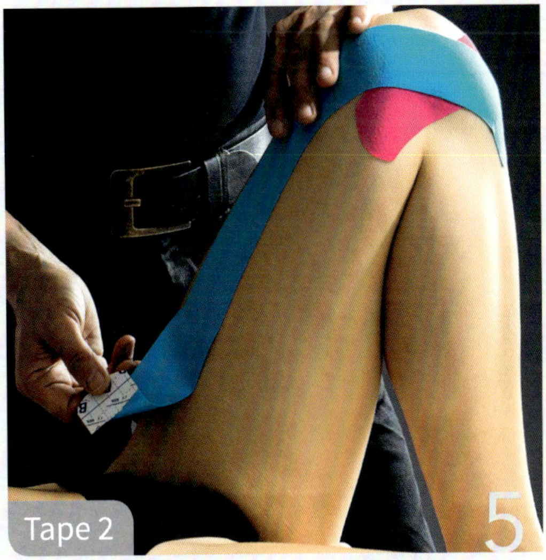

Tapelänge abmessen (Länge siehe Foto)

Gauge tape length (for length, see photo)

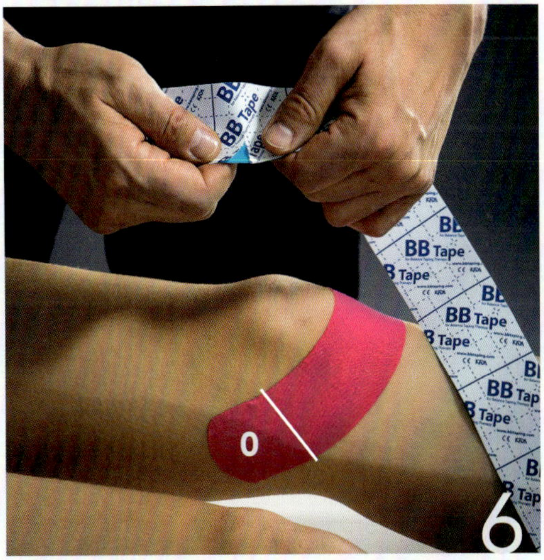

Nach 10 cm Länge das Trennpapier einreißen, Knie leicht anbeugen

Tear the backing paper at a length of 10 cm, bend the knee a little

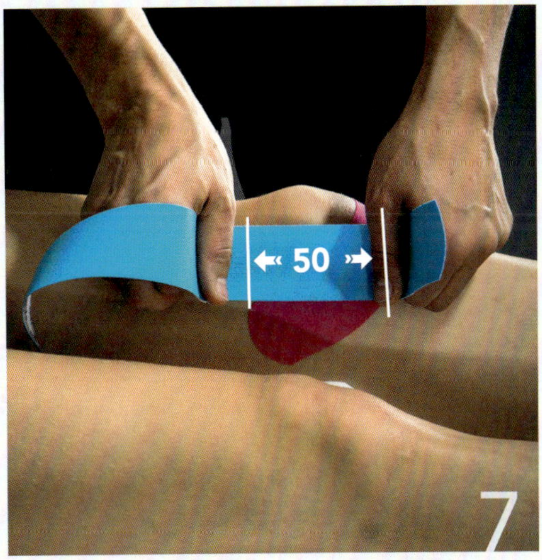

Tape auf die Innenseite des Kniegelenkes kleben

Affix tape to the inside of the knee

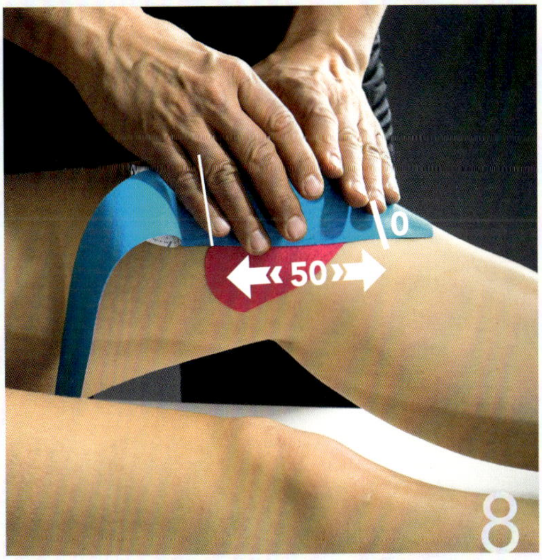

Unteres Tapeende aufkleben

Affix lower end of tape

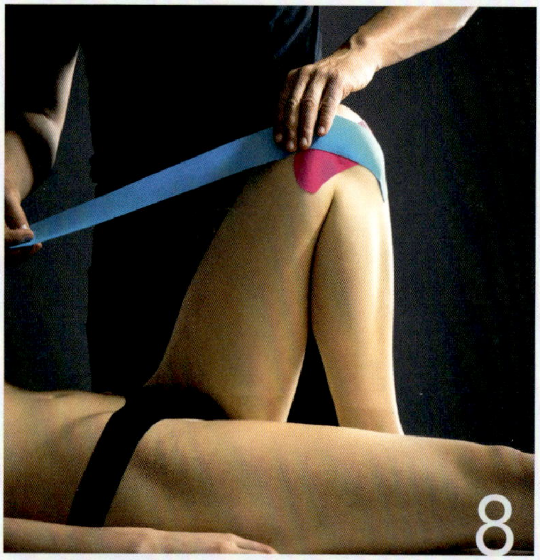

Jetzt Muskeln vordehnen

Now pre-stretch the muscles

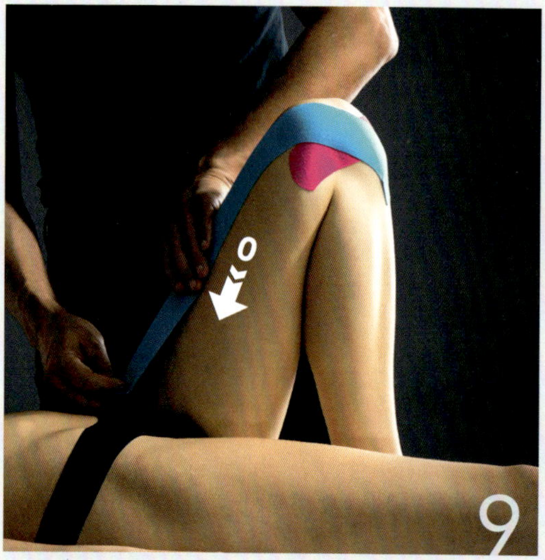

Tapezügel um die Muskeln bis zur Leiste (Innenseite) aufkleben

Affix tape tails around the muscles as far as the groin (inner)

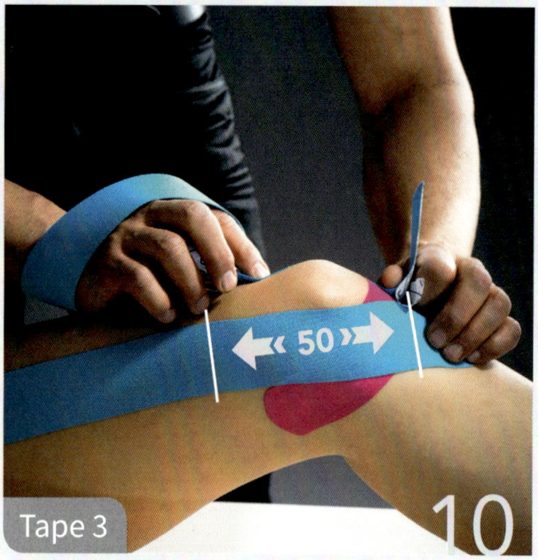

2. Tapezügel außen wie Innenseite kleben

Affix 2nd tape tail on the outside as for the inside

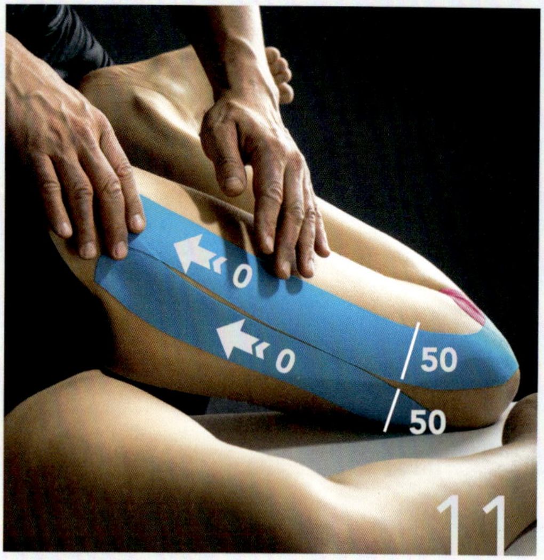

Tape anreiben

Rub down the tape

Halswirbelsäule Basis Tape

Cervical spine base tape

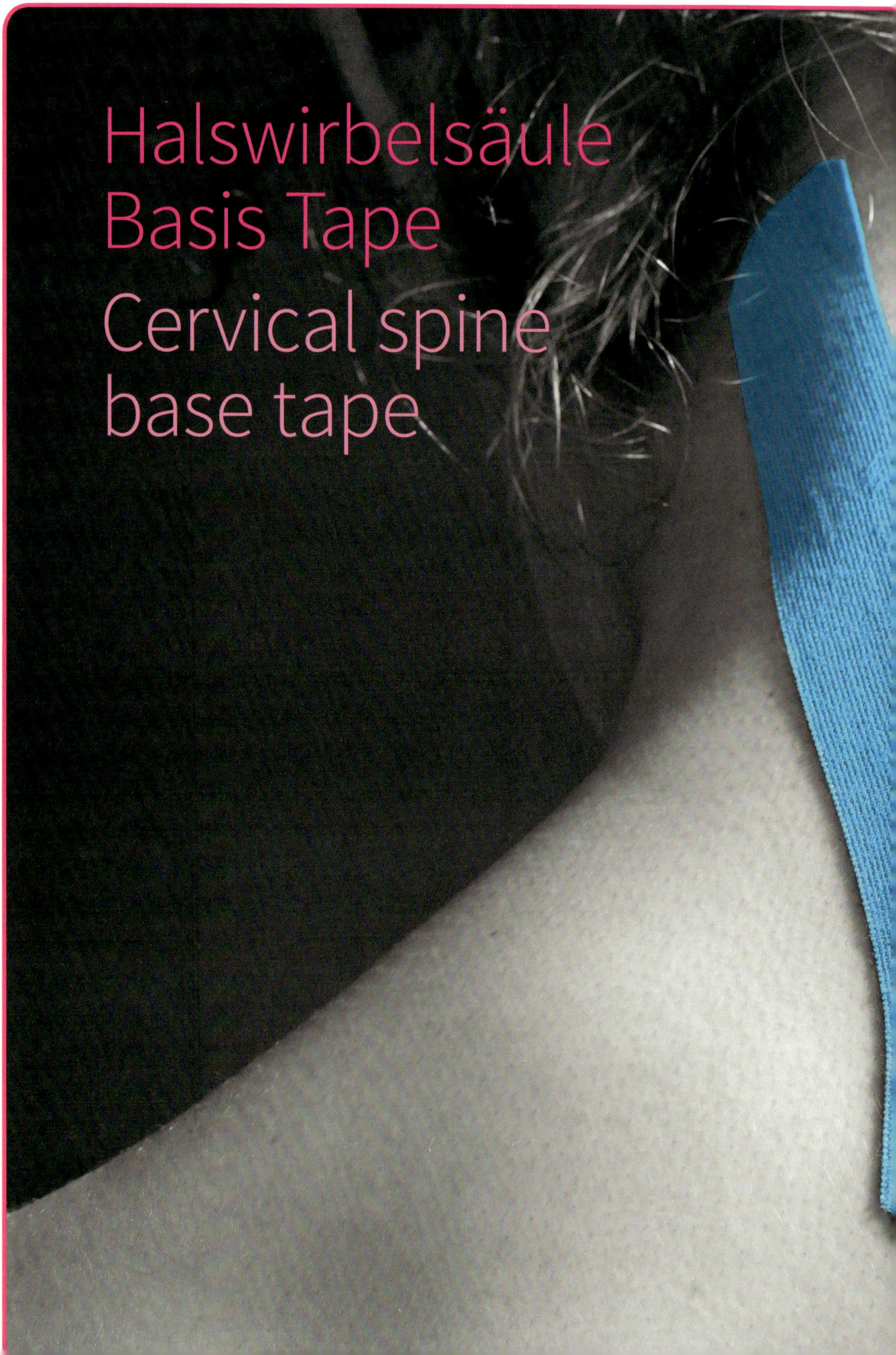

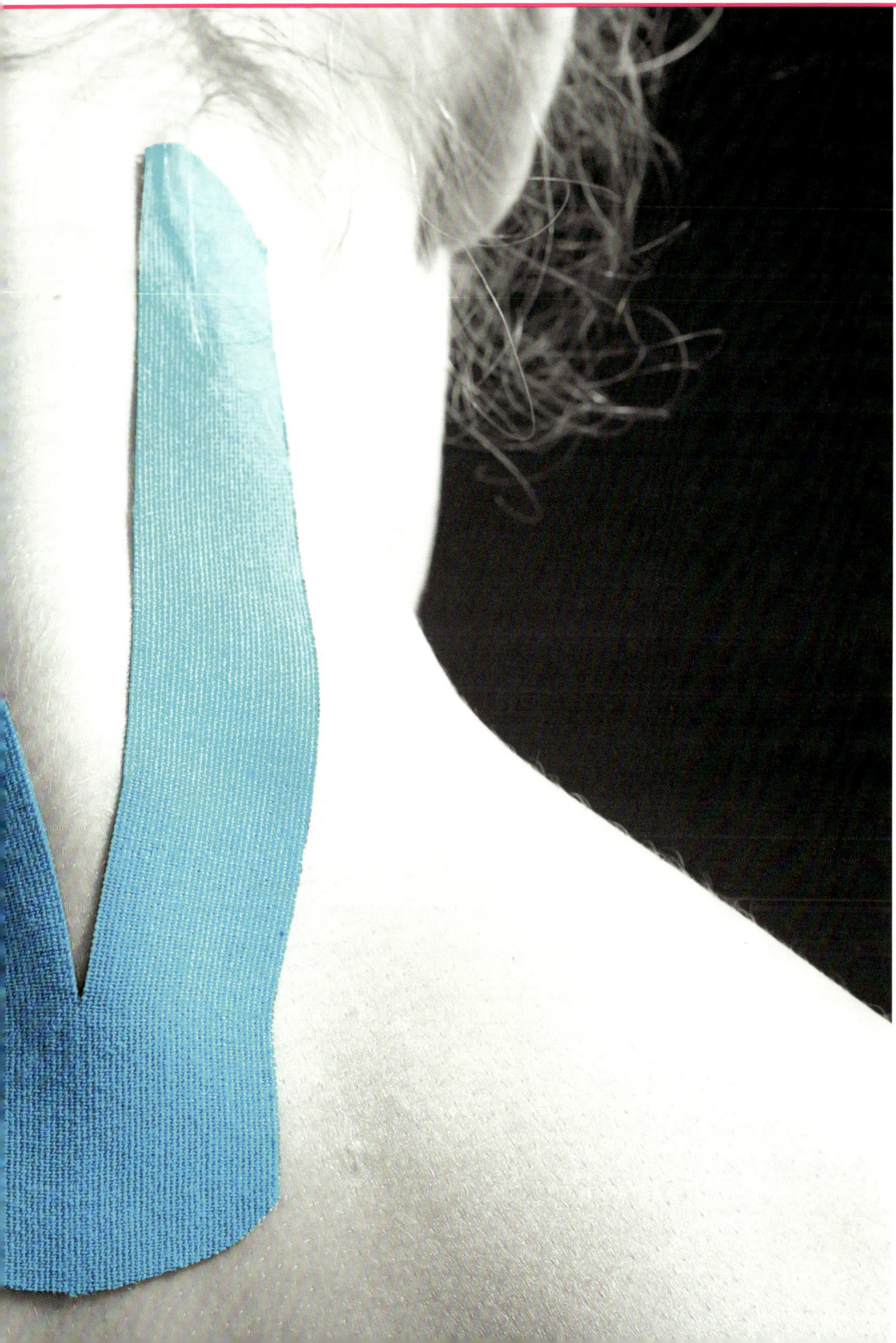

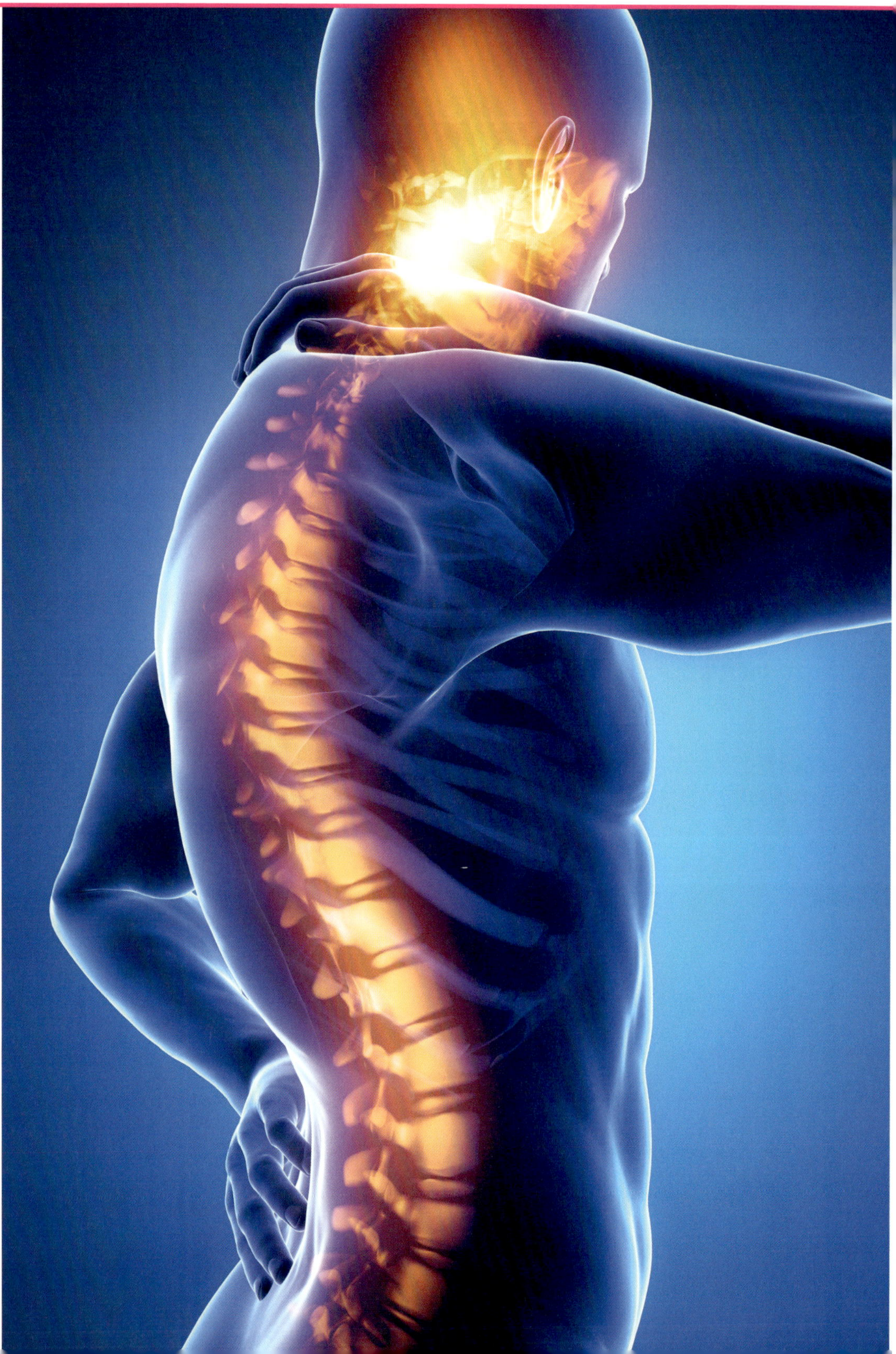

Halswirbelsäule
Cervical spine

Hinweise

Das Tape wird angelegt bei:

- Beschwerden an der Halswirbelsäule
- Nackenverspannungen
- Schleudertrauma

Advice

The tape is applied for:

- Discomfort in the cervical spine
- Neck tension
- Whiplash

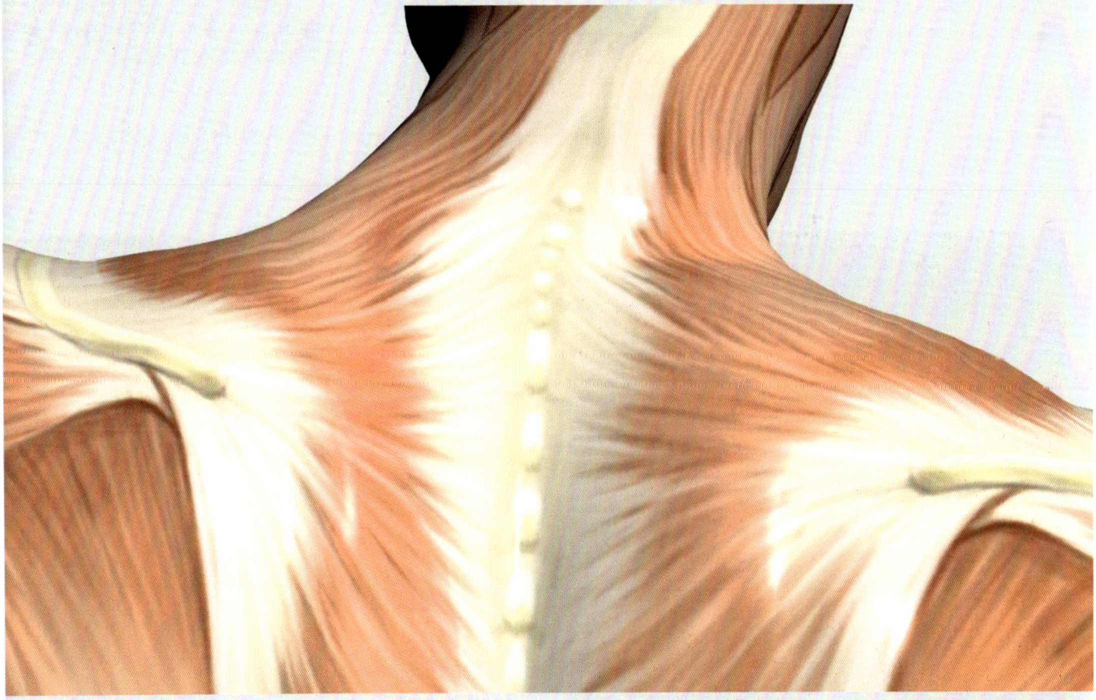

Bitte nutzen Sie die Gitterpflaster zur Wirkungsverbesserung vor jeder Anwendung. Einfach auf die Schmerzpunkte kleben

Please use the cross-tapes to improve the effect prior to each application Simply affix to the painful spots

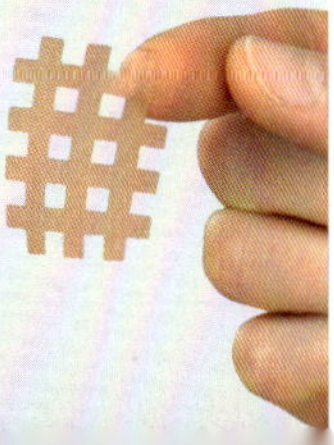

Halswirbelsäule Basis Tape

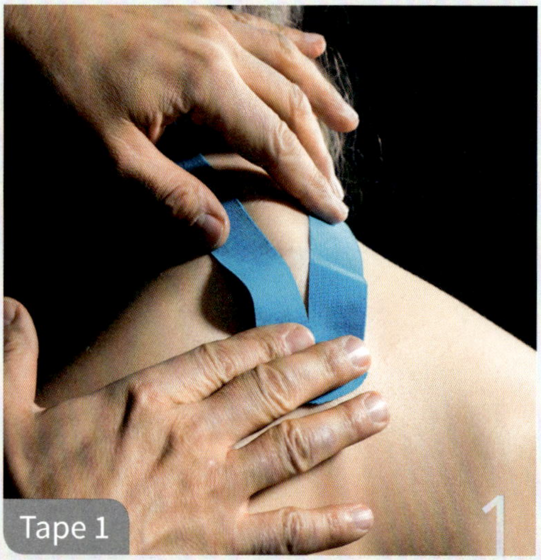

Tapelänge abmessen – vom Haaransatz bis zum 1. Brustwirbel (siehe Foto)

Gauge tape length – from hairline to the first thoracic (see photo)

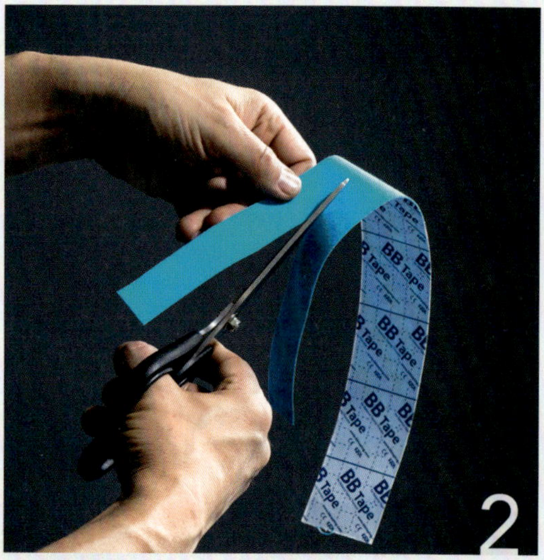

Tape bis auf 5 cm der Länge halbieren

Halve tape lengthways, leaving 5 cm at the end

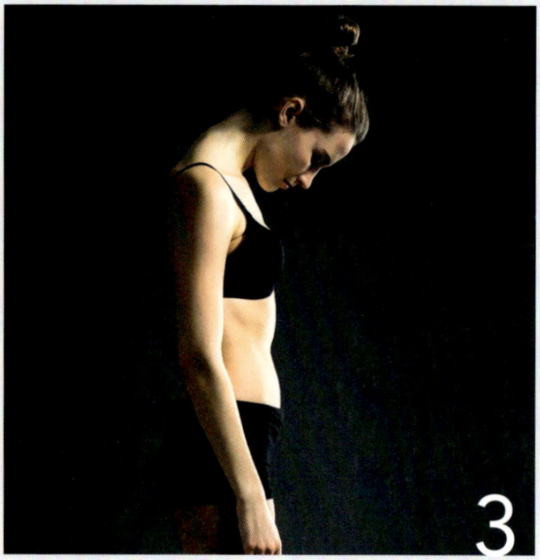

Muskeln vordehnen

Pre-stretch the muscles

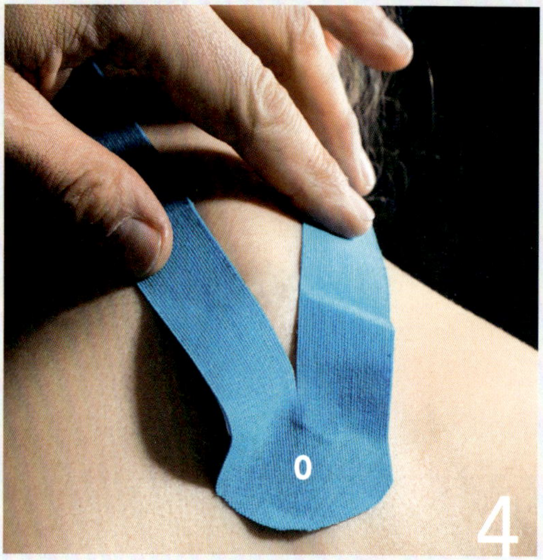

Tapebasis auf dem 1. Brustwirbel aufkleben

Affix base tape to the 1st thoracic vertebra

Cervical spine base tape

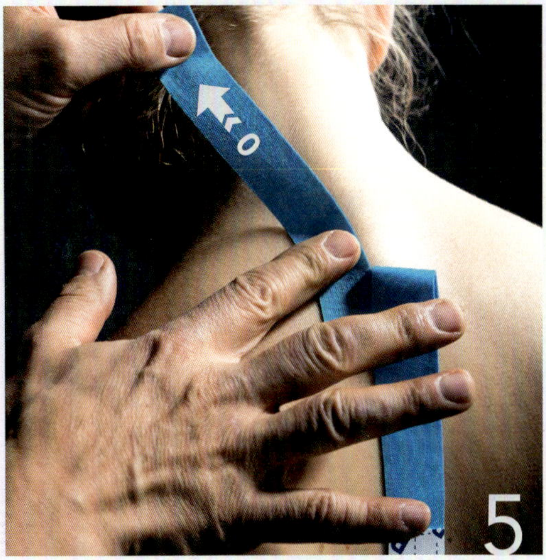

Tapezügel um die Dornfortsätze anlegen (nicht in die Haare!)

Position tape tails around the spinous (not in the hair!)

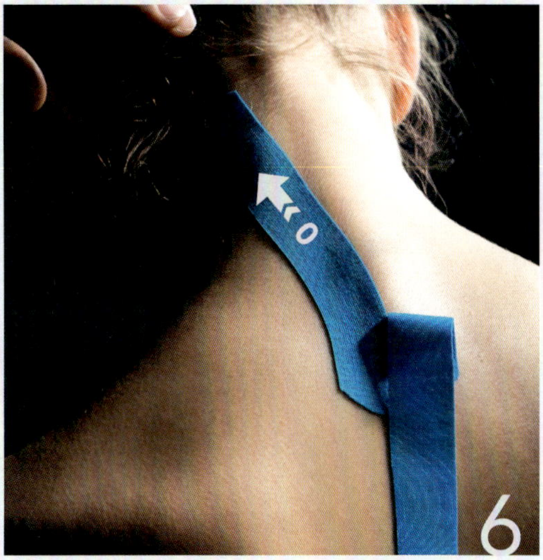

Tapezügel auf die Muskeln anlegen

Position tape tails on the muscles

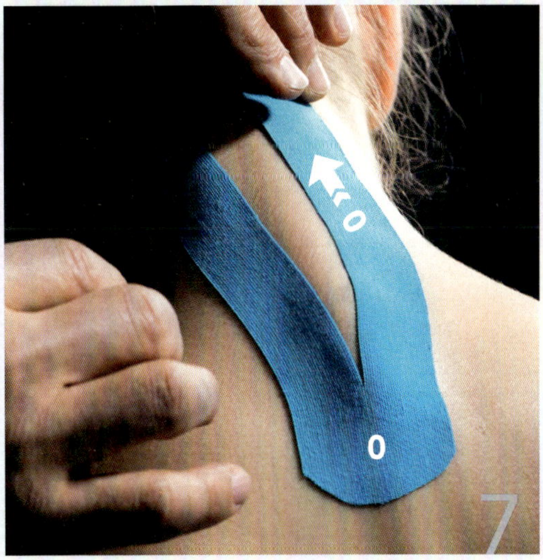

Tapezügel auf die Muskeln anlegen

Position tape tails on the muscles

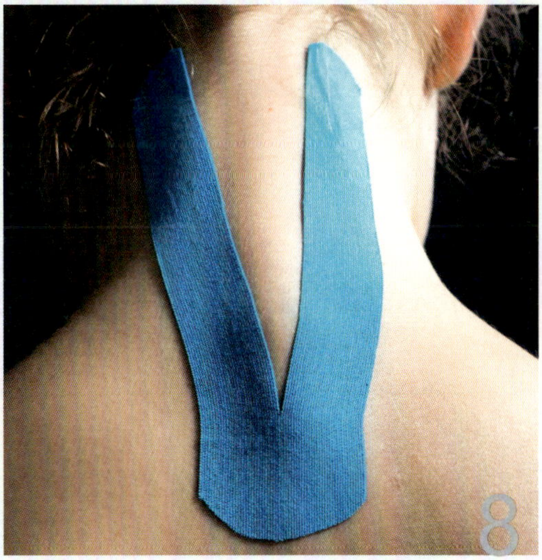

Tape anreiben

Rub down the tape

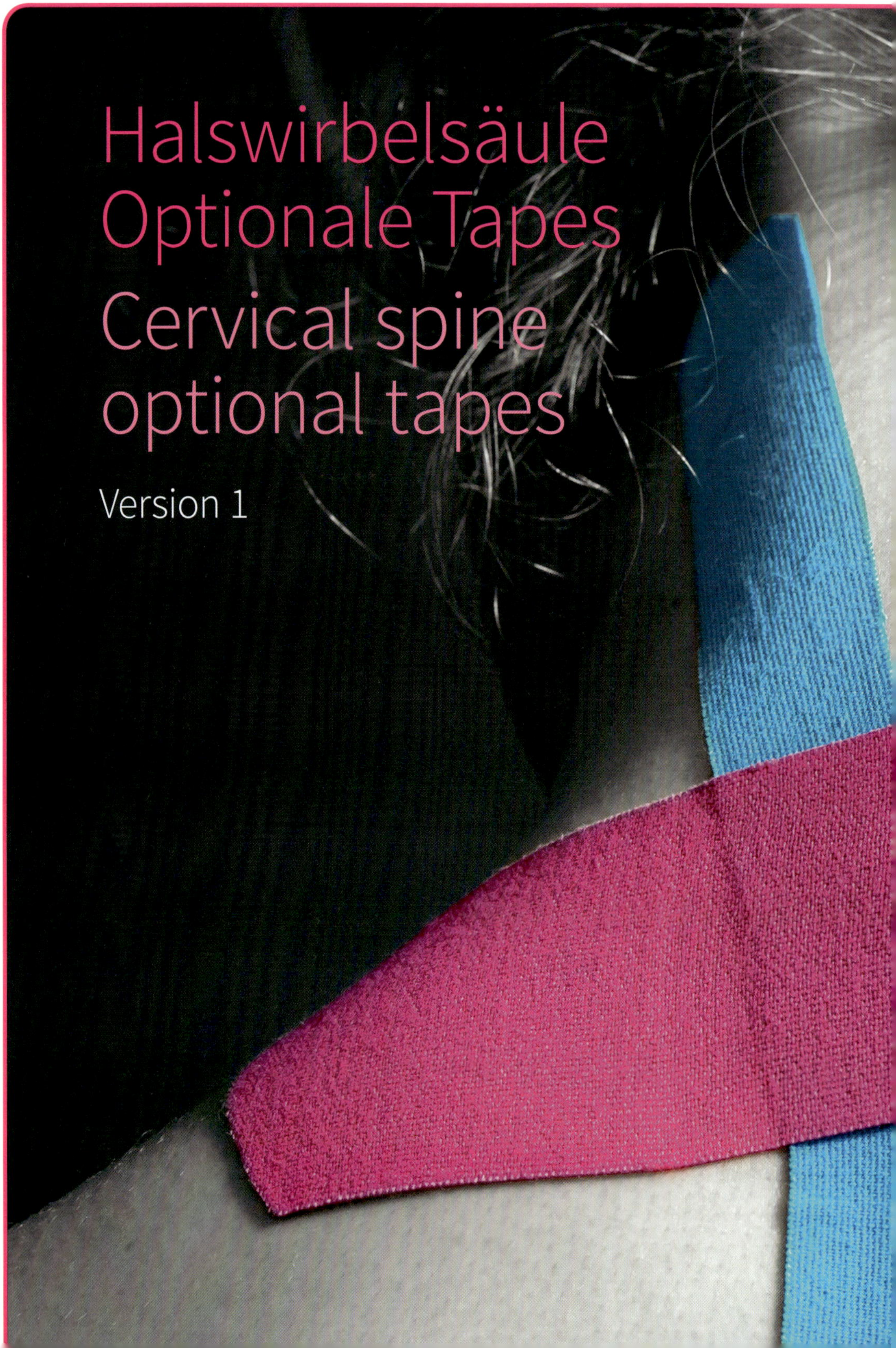

Halswirbelsäule Optionale Tapes

Cervical spine optional tapes

Version 1

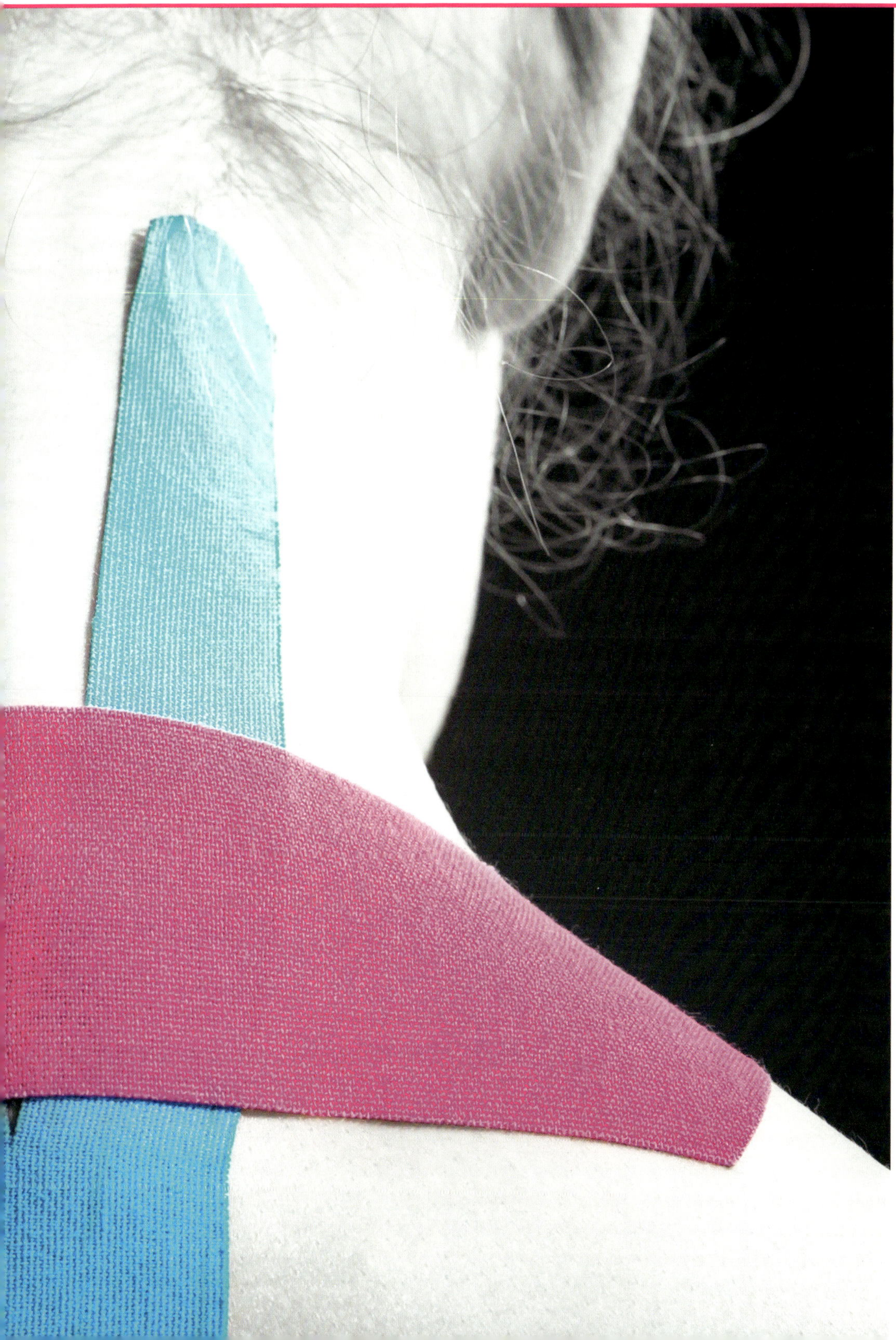

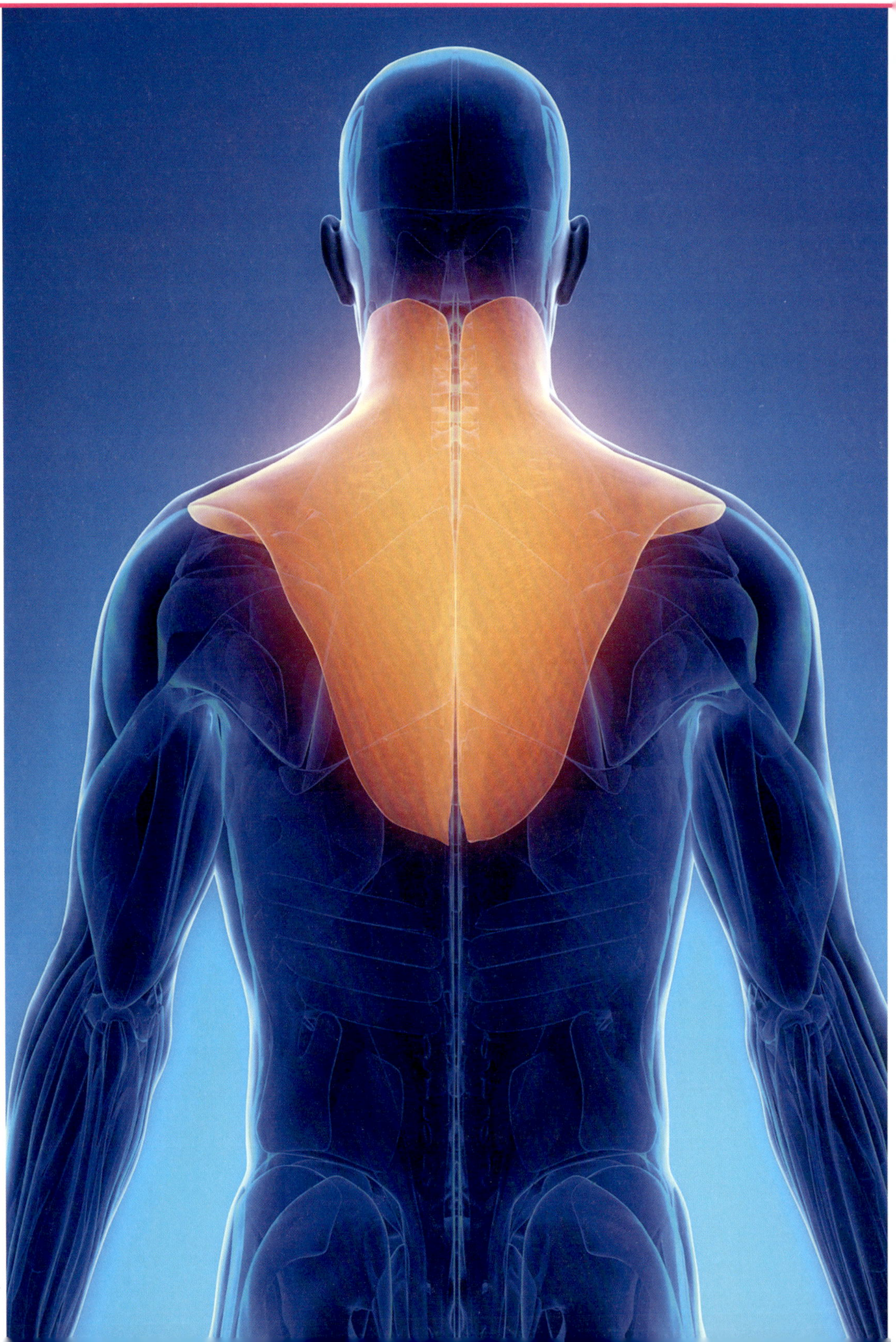

Halswirbelsäule Optionale Tapes
Cervical spine optional tapes

Hinweise

Das Tape wird angelegt bei:

- Beschwerden an der Halswirbelsäule
- Starken Nackenverspannungen
- Einschränkungen beim Kopf drehen
- Beschwerden beim Blick über die Schulter nach hinten
- Beschwerden, welche bis zum Schulterblatt ausstrahlen
- Schleudertrauma

Advice

The tape is applied for:

- Discomfort in the cervical spine
- Severe neck tension
- Restrictions when turning the head
- Discomfort when looking backwards over the shoulders
- Discomfort radiating as far as the shoulder blade
- Whiplash

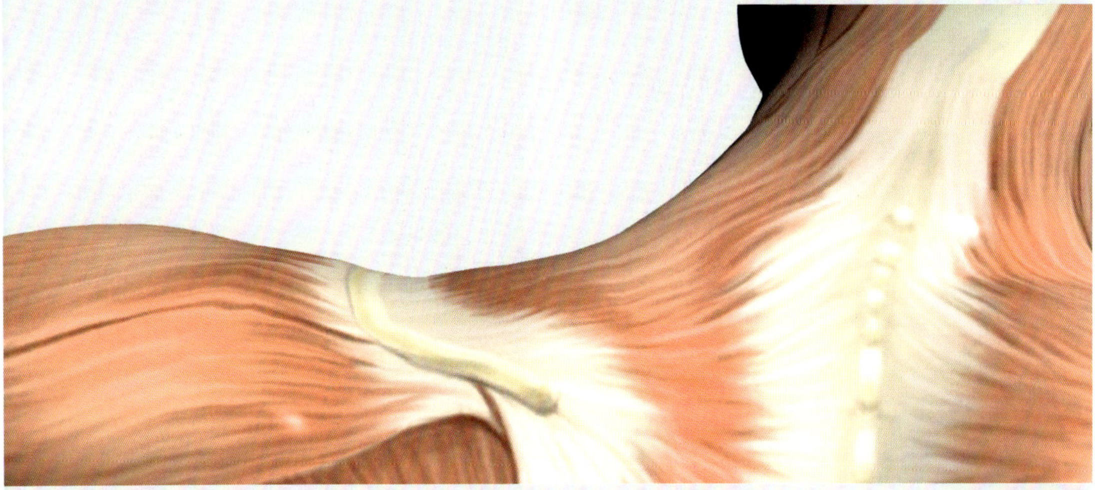

Bitte nutzen Sie die Gitterpflaster zur Wirkungsverbesserung vor jeder Anwendung. Einfach auf die Schmerzpunkte kleben

Please use the cross-tapes to improve the effect prior to each application Simply affix to the painful spots

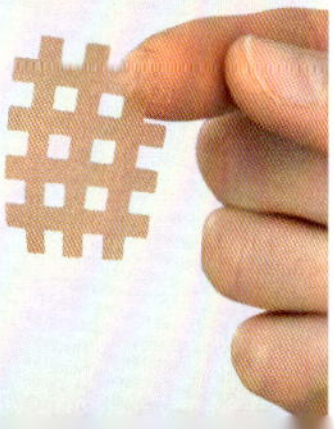

Halswirbelsäule Optionales Tape

Version 1

Dieser Tape entlastet zusätzlich die Halswirbelsäule.

Sollte sich der Patient in den ersten 15 min mit dem Tape unwohl fühlen, bitte dieses Tape wieder entfernen. (Darf der Patient auch jederzeit selbst tun)

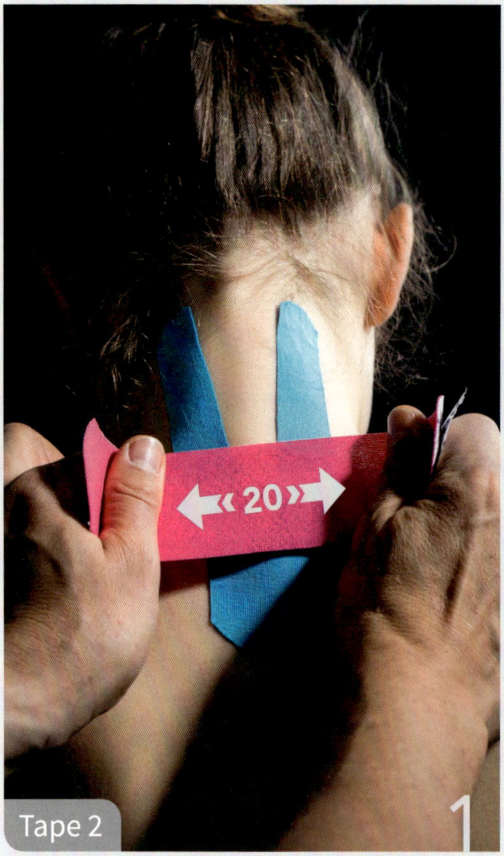

In Höhe der letzten Halswirbel platzieren. Tape nur aufkleben, wenn es sich um eine Blockade handelt

Position at the level of the last cervical vertebra. Affix tape only if there is a blockage

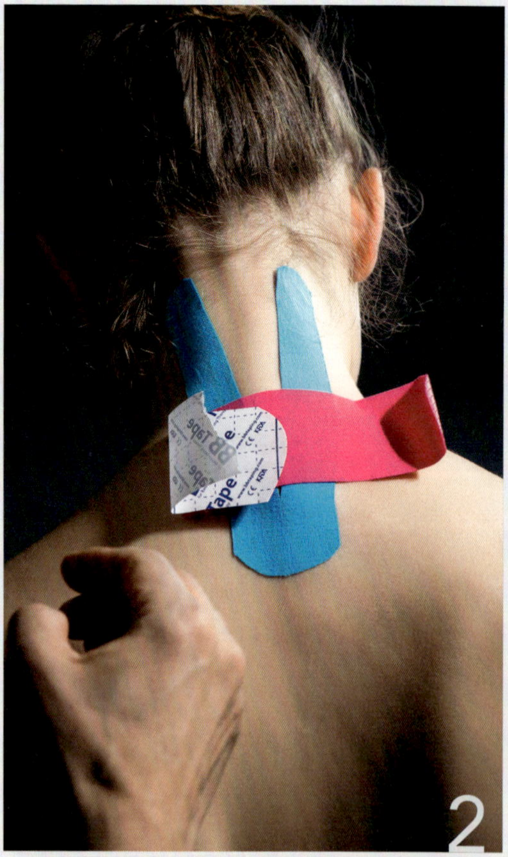

Enden nicht mit aufkleben

Do not affix the ends

Cervical spine optional tape

version 1

This tape relieves the cervical spine additionally.

If the patient feels uncomfortable with the tape within the first 15 minutes, please remove this tape. (Patients can also do this themselves at any time)

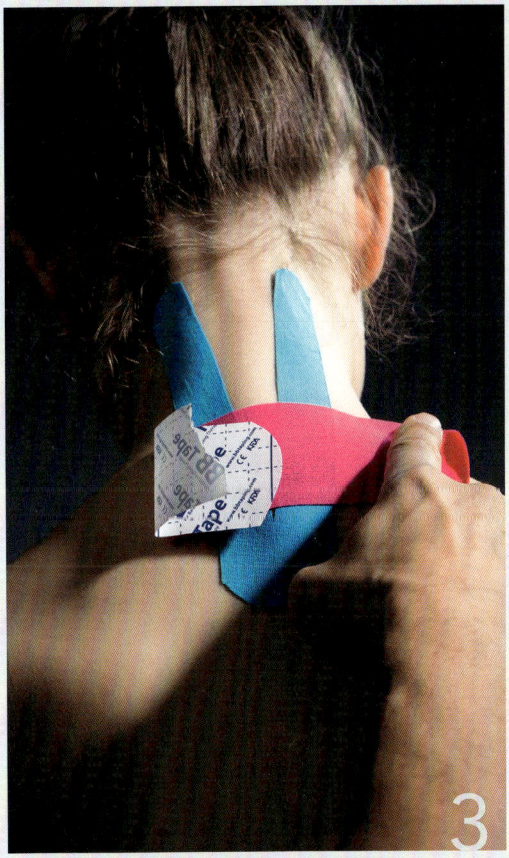

Enden ohne Zug aufkleben

Affix ends without stretch

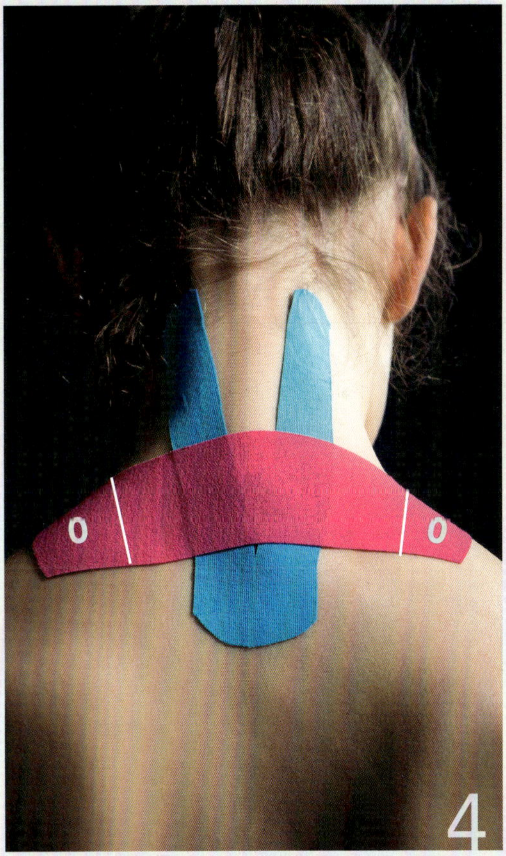

Fertig!

That's it!

Halswirbelsäule Optionale Tapes

Cervical spine optional tapes

Version 2

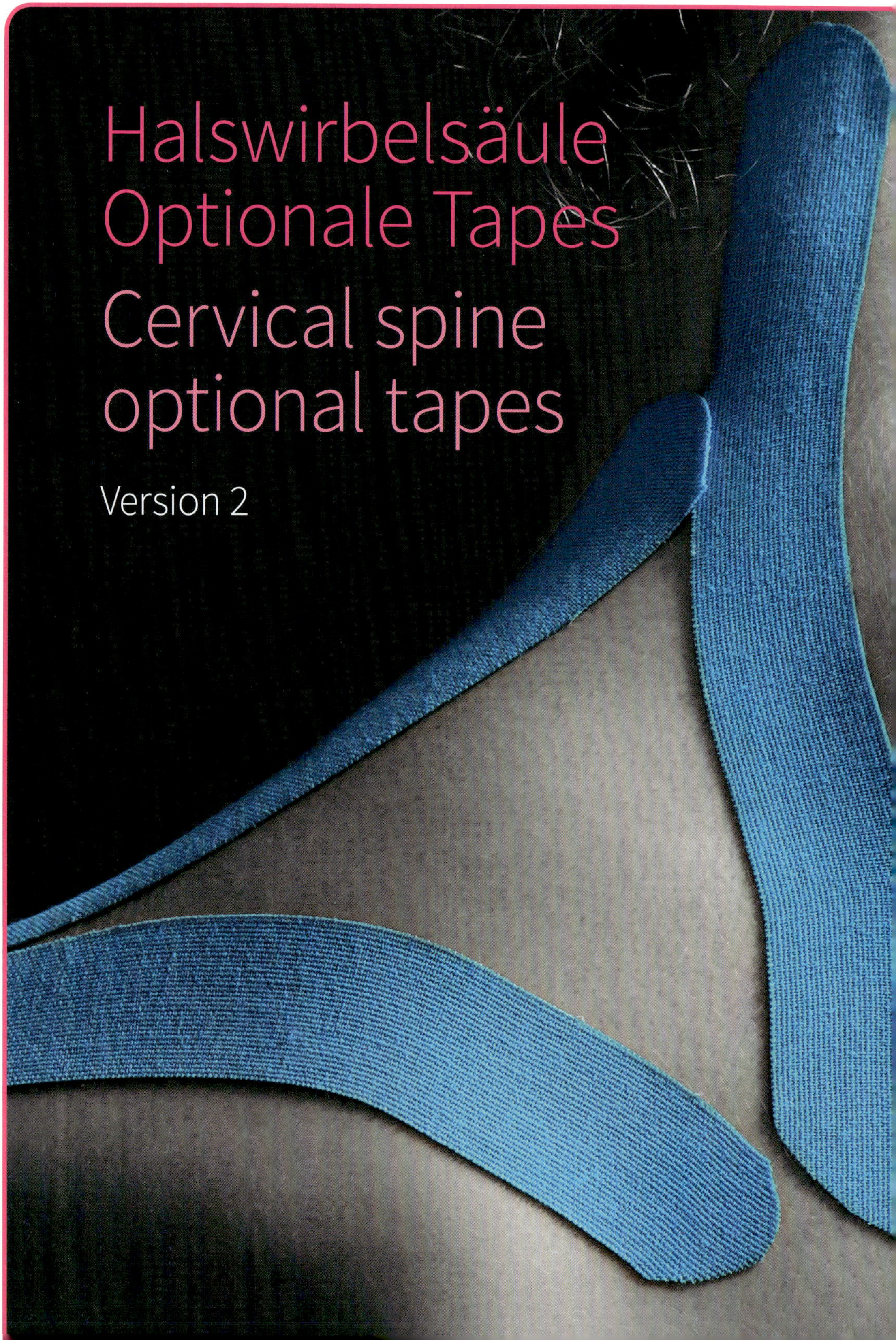

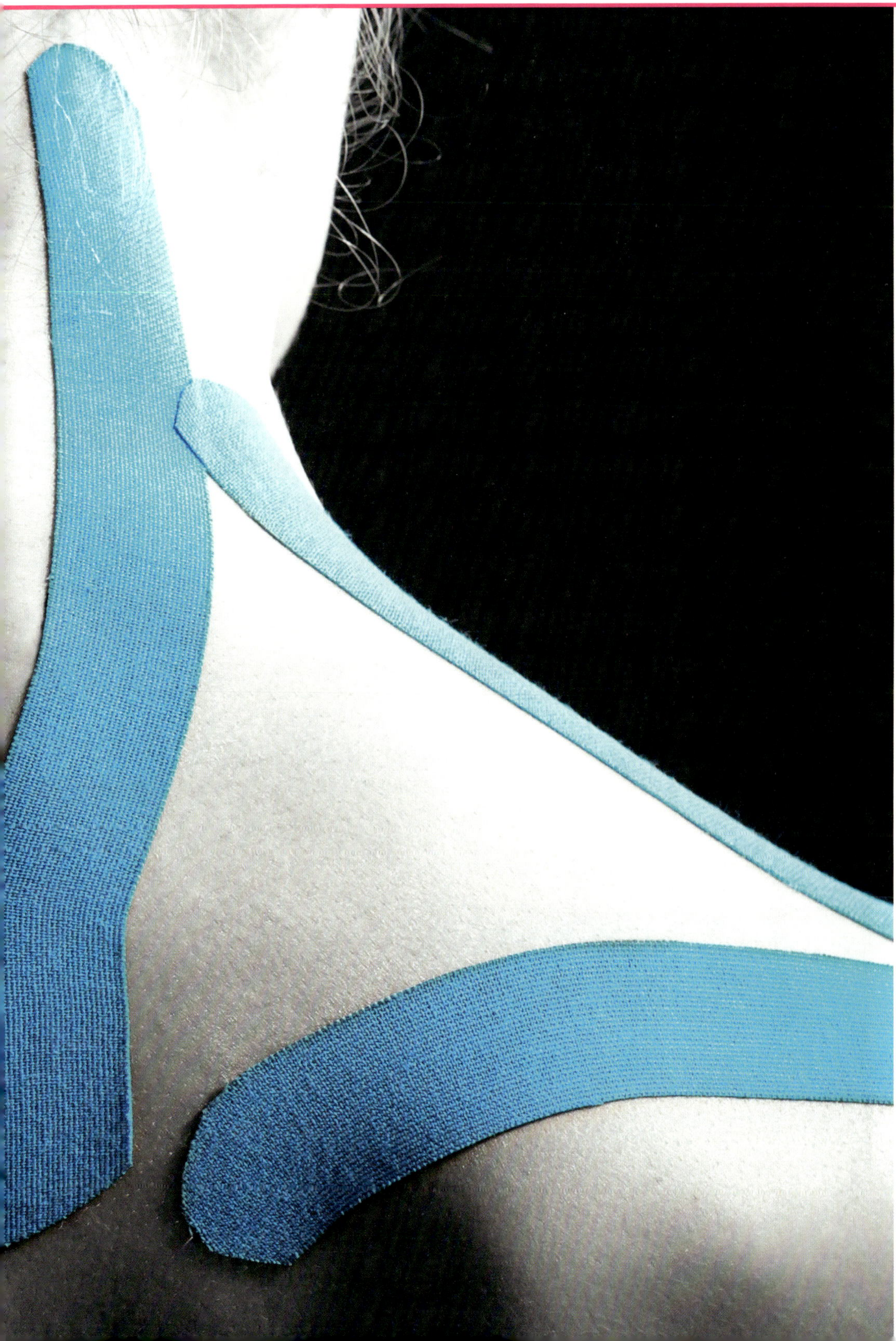

Halswirbelsäule Optionales Tape

Version 2 **Dieser Tape wird zusätzlich zu Tape Version 1 geklebt**

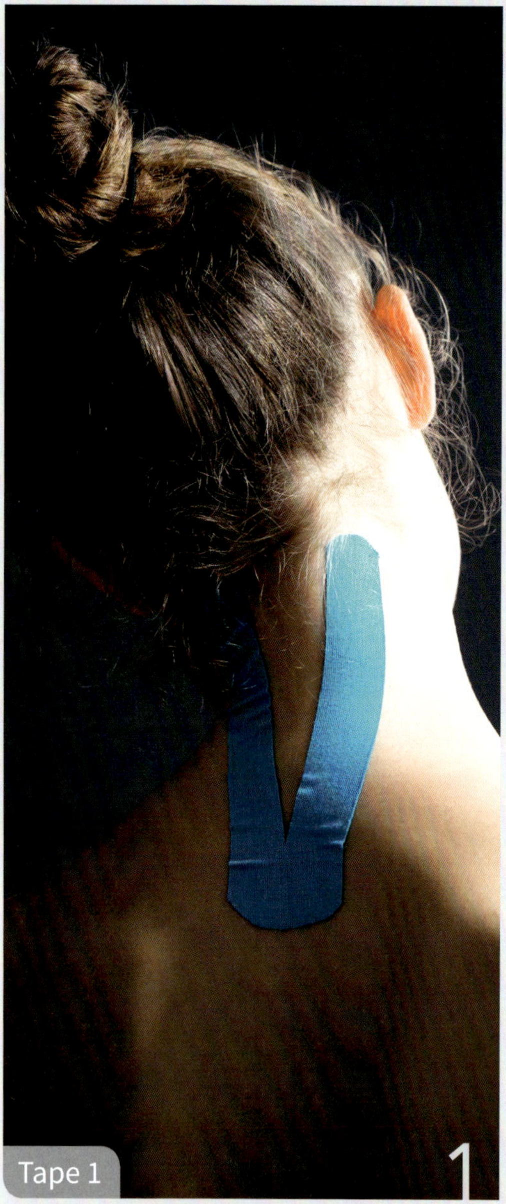

Muskeln vordehnen

Pre-stretch the muscles

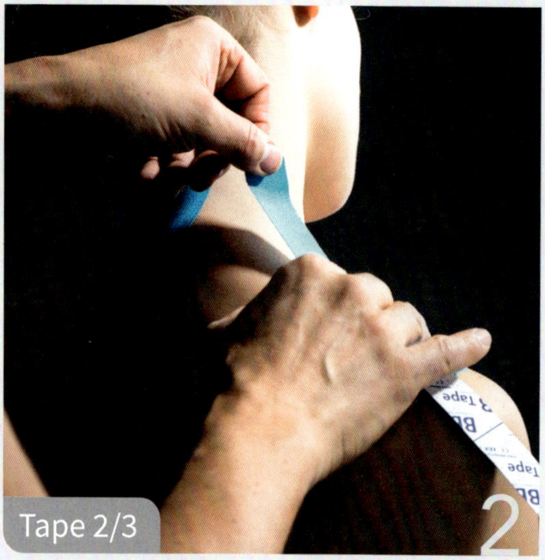

Tapelänge abmessen, vom ACG (Acromioclavicular-Gelenk) bis Mitte Halslänge

Gauge tape length, from acromioclavicular joint up to the mid of neck

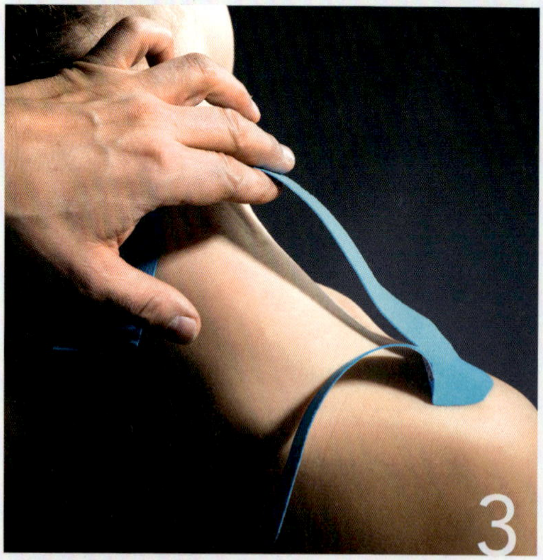

Tapezügel einschneiden und Basis auf das AC-Gelenk aufkleben

Cut the tape tails and affix the base to the AC joint

Cervical spine optional tape

version 2 This tape will be applied additionally to tape version 1

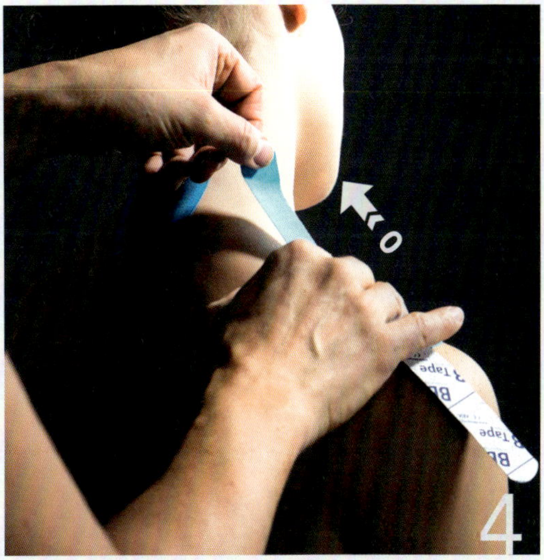

Tapezügel Richtung Ohrläppchen anlegen

Position tape tail in direction to ear tip

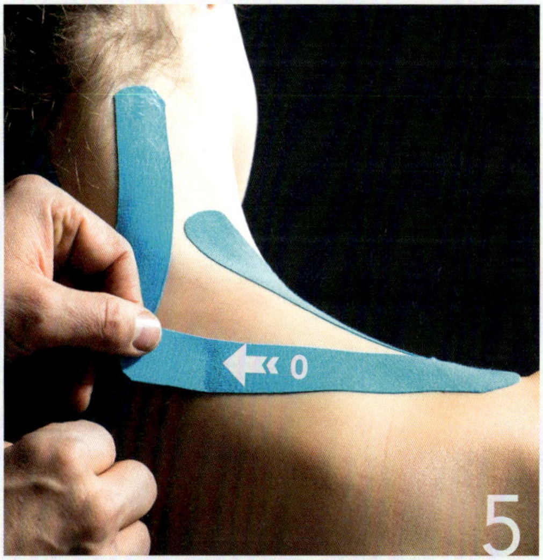

Tapezügel um das Schulterblatt anlegen

Position tape tail around the shoulder blade

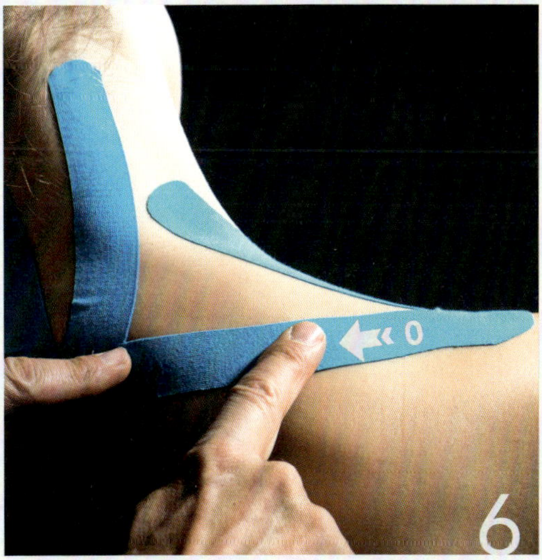

Tapezügel ohne Zug anlegen

Position tape tails without stretch

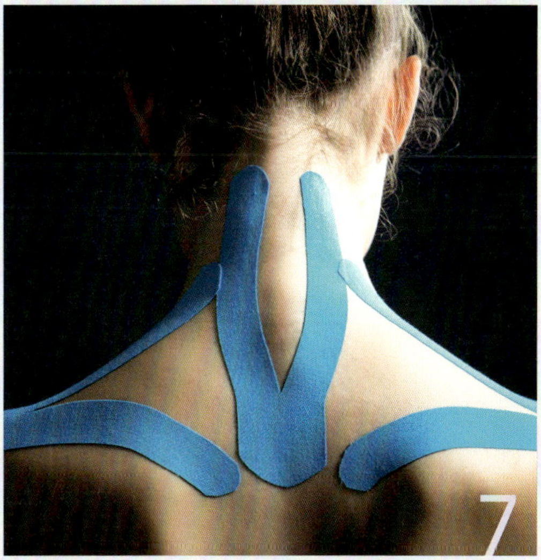

Fertig!

That's it!

Achillessehne Basis Tape

Achilles tendon base tape

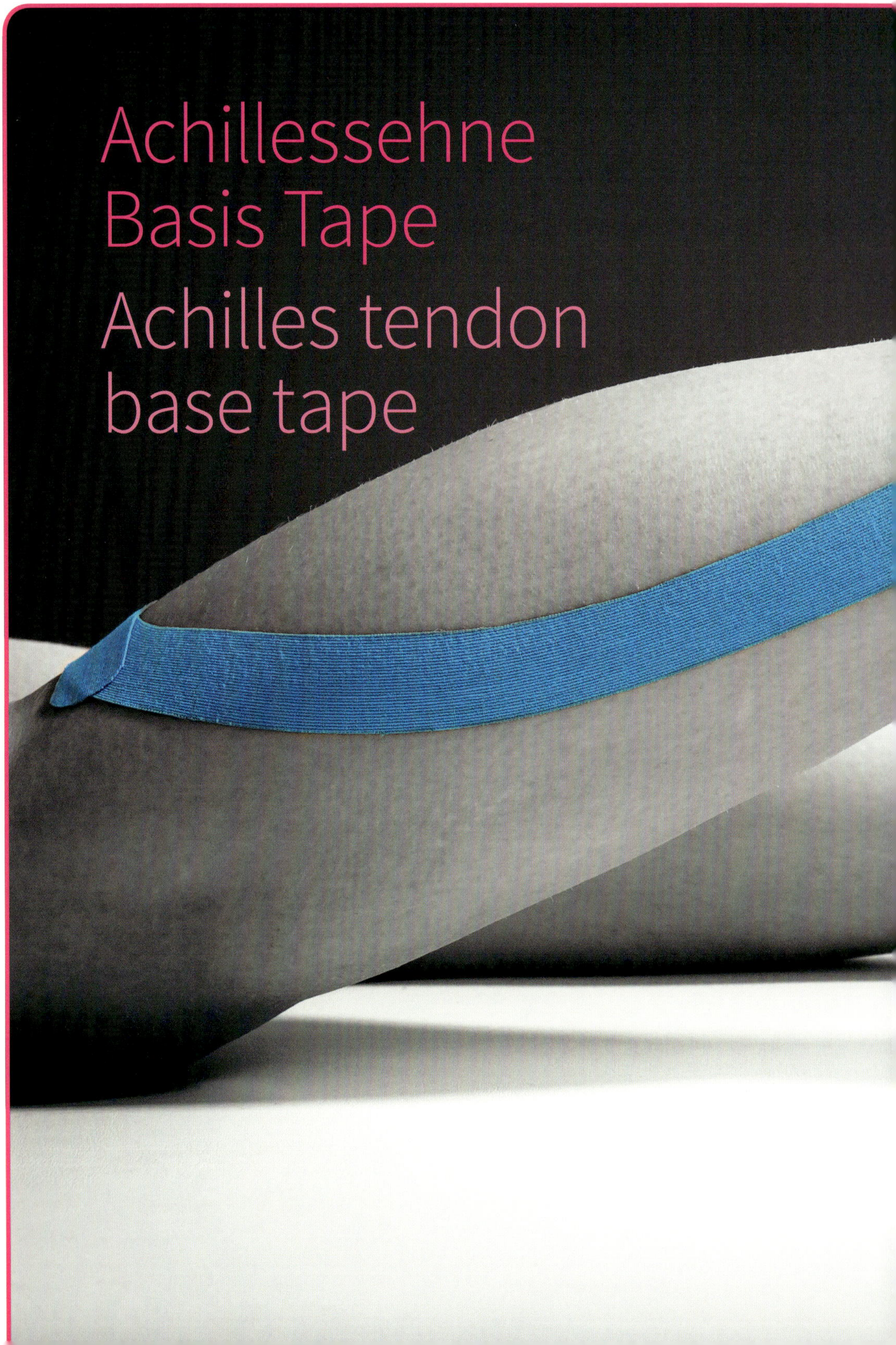

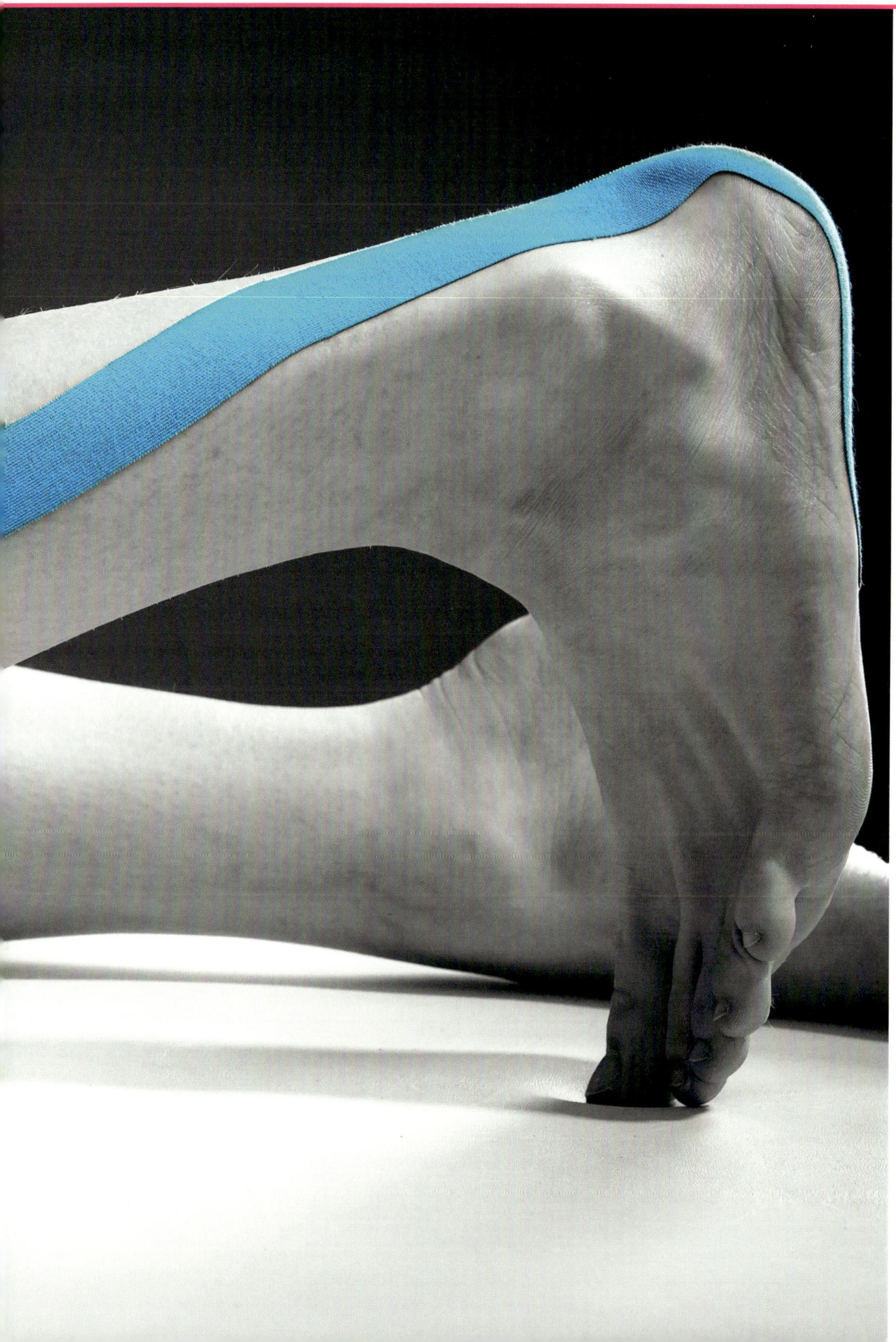

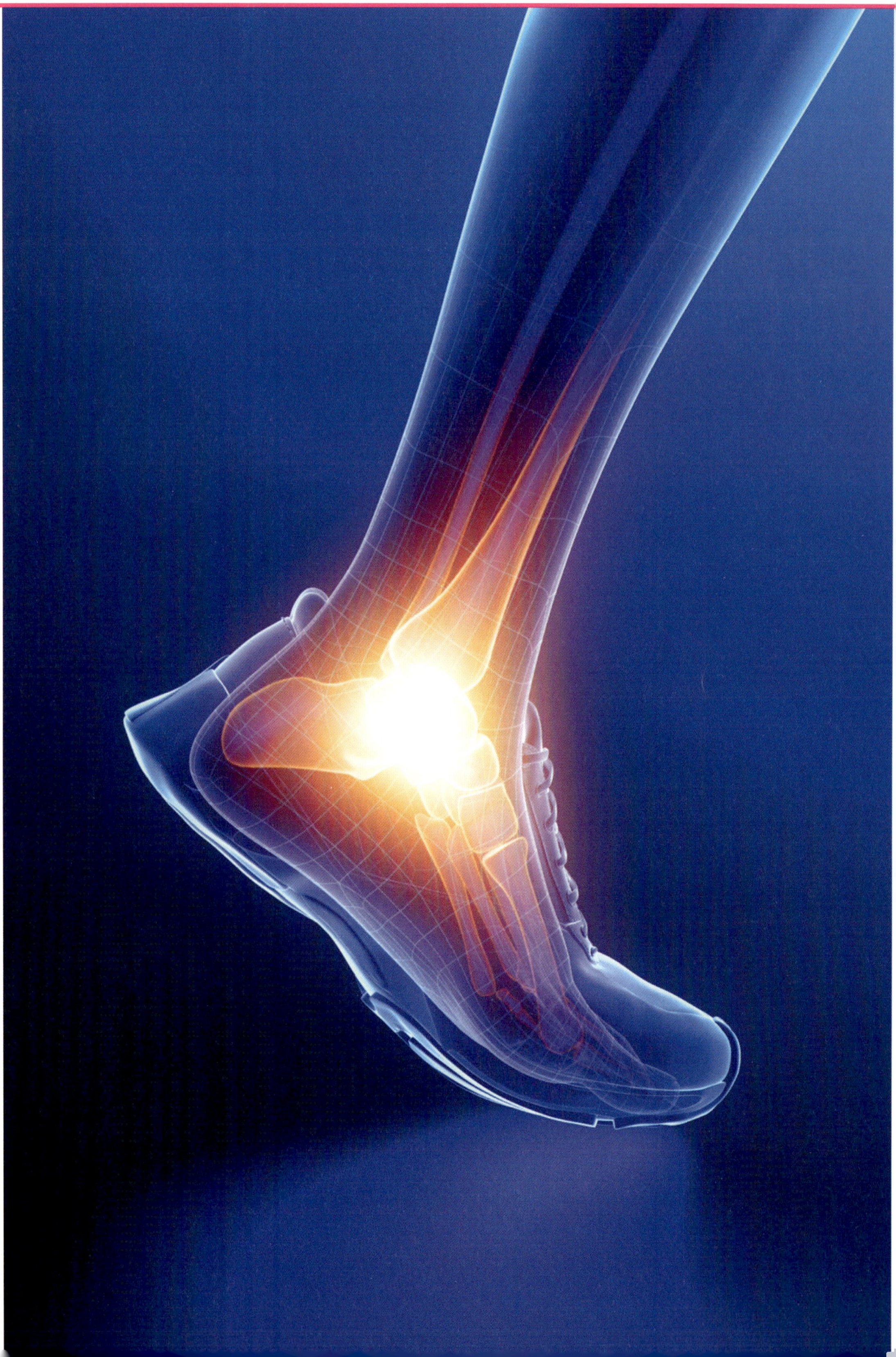

Achillessehne
Achilles tendon

Hinweise

Das Tape wird angelegt bei:

- bei allen Beschwerden an der Achillessehne
- nach Verletzung
- nach OP
- Belastungsbeschwerden
- Entzündung
- Vernarbung

Dieser Tape ist ausreichend zur Versorgung von Beschwerden an der Achillessehne.

Advice

The tape is applied for:

- all discomfort at the Achilles tendon
- following injury
- following surgery
- weight-bearing discomfort
- inflammation
- scar tissue

This tape is sufficient to treat discomfort at the Achilles tendon.

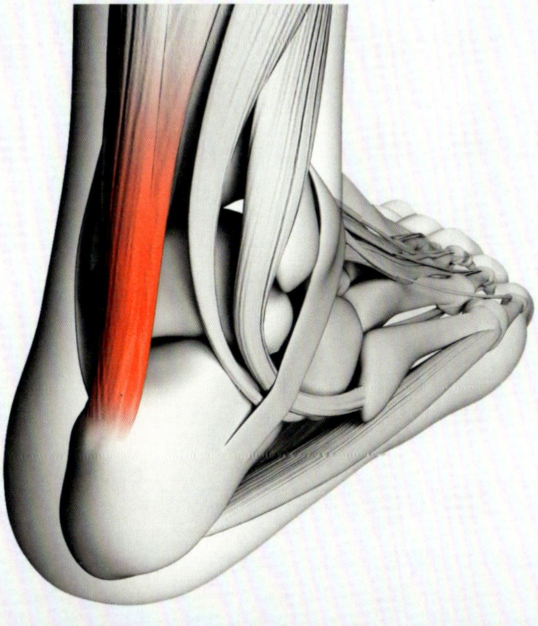

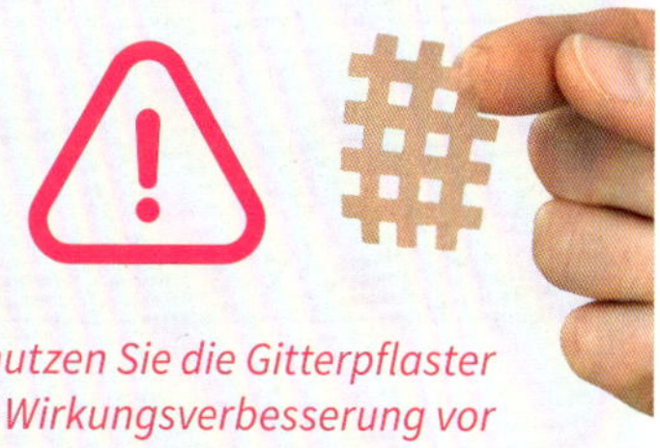

Bitte nutzen Sie die Gitterpflaster zur Wirkungsverbesserung vor jeder Anwendung. Einfach auf die Schmerzpunkte kleben

Please use the cross-tapes to improve the effect prior to each application Simply affix to the painful spots

Achillessehne – Basis Tape

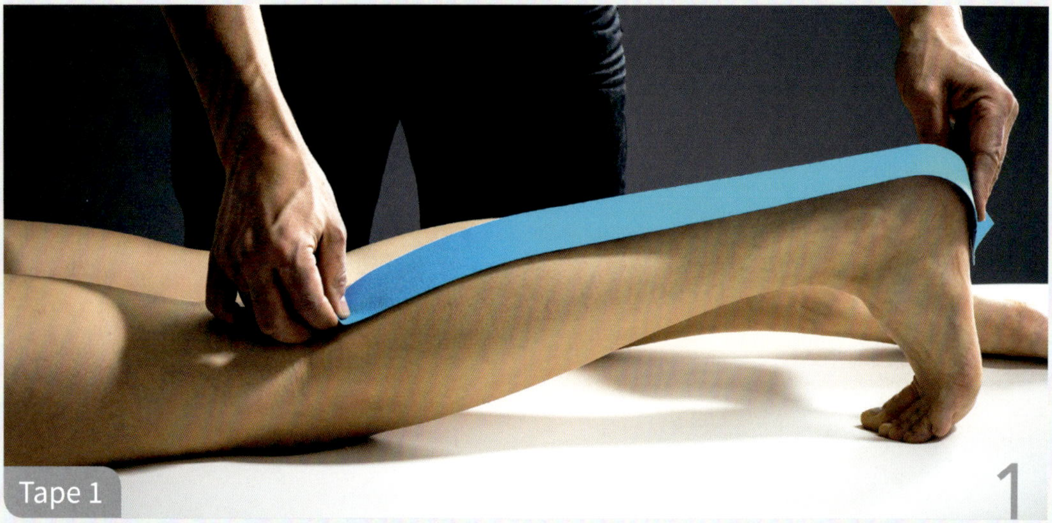

Tapelänge: Von der Fußsohle bis zur Kniekehle. Bitte nicht in die Kniekehle kleben!

Tape length: from the sole of the foot to the back of the knee. Please do not affix to the back of the knee!

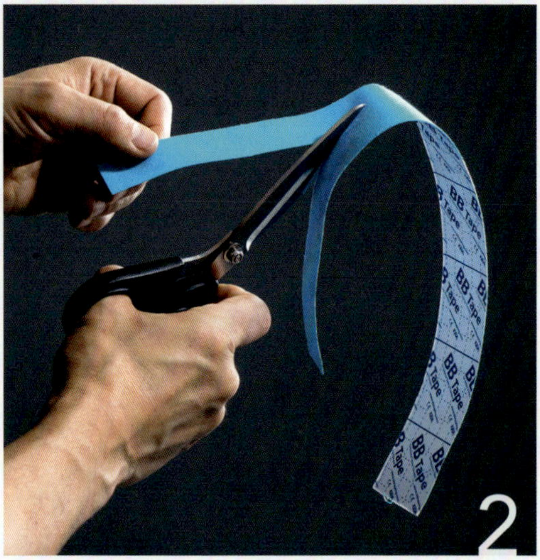

Tapezügel bis auf 5 cm halbieren

Halve tape tails lengthways, leaving 5 cm at the end

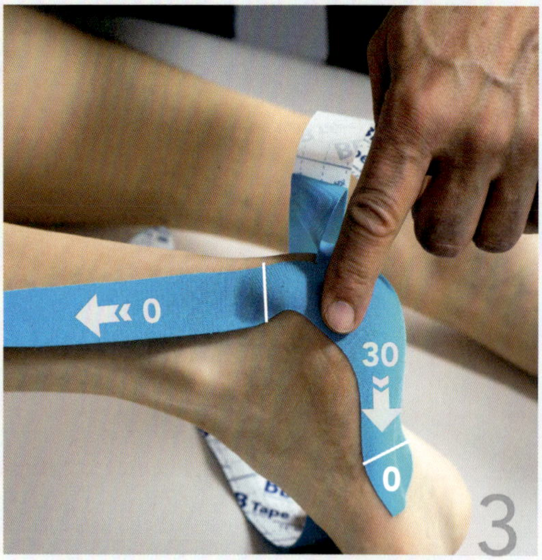

Tape mit wenig Zug über der Ferse und ohne Zug unter dem Fuß aufkleben, Zehenspitzen aufstellen

Affix tape over the heel with a little stretch and underneath the foot without stretch; tuck the toes under

Achilles tendon – base tape

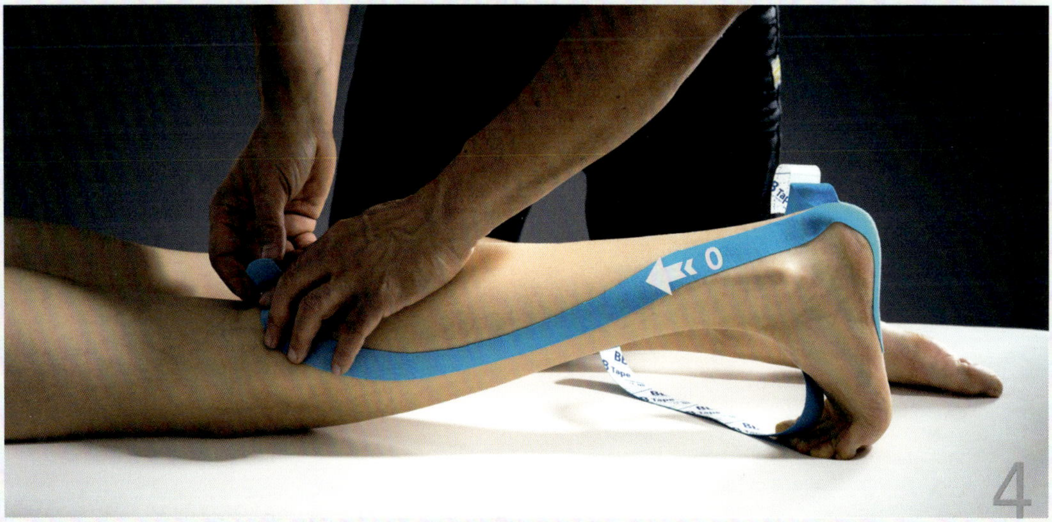

Tapezügel 1 um den Muskelbauch der Wade aussen aufkleben

Affix the tape tail 1 around the outside of the calf muscle belly

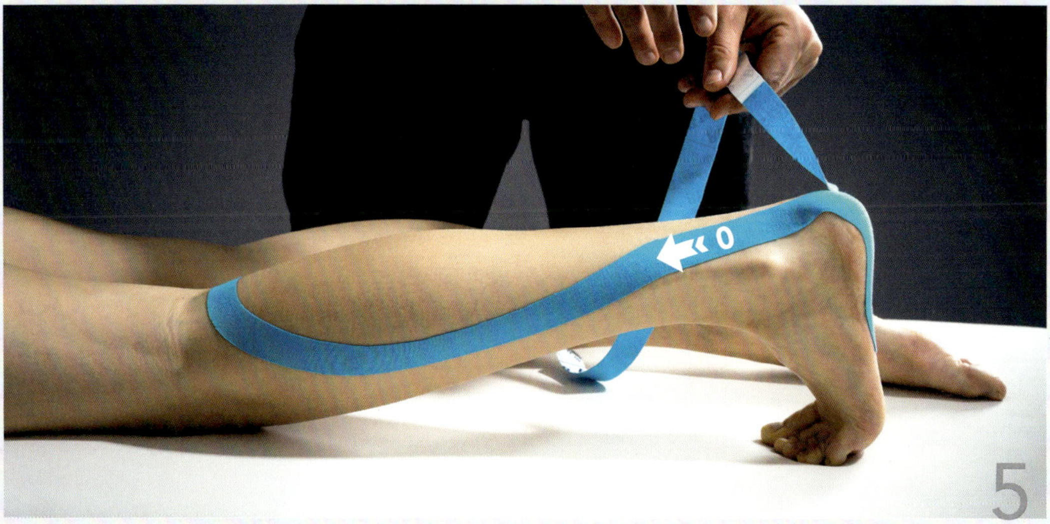

Tapezügel 2 um den Muskelbauch der Wade innen aufkleben

Affix the tape tail 2 around the inside of the calf muscle belly

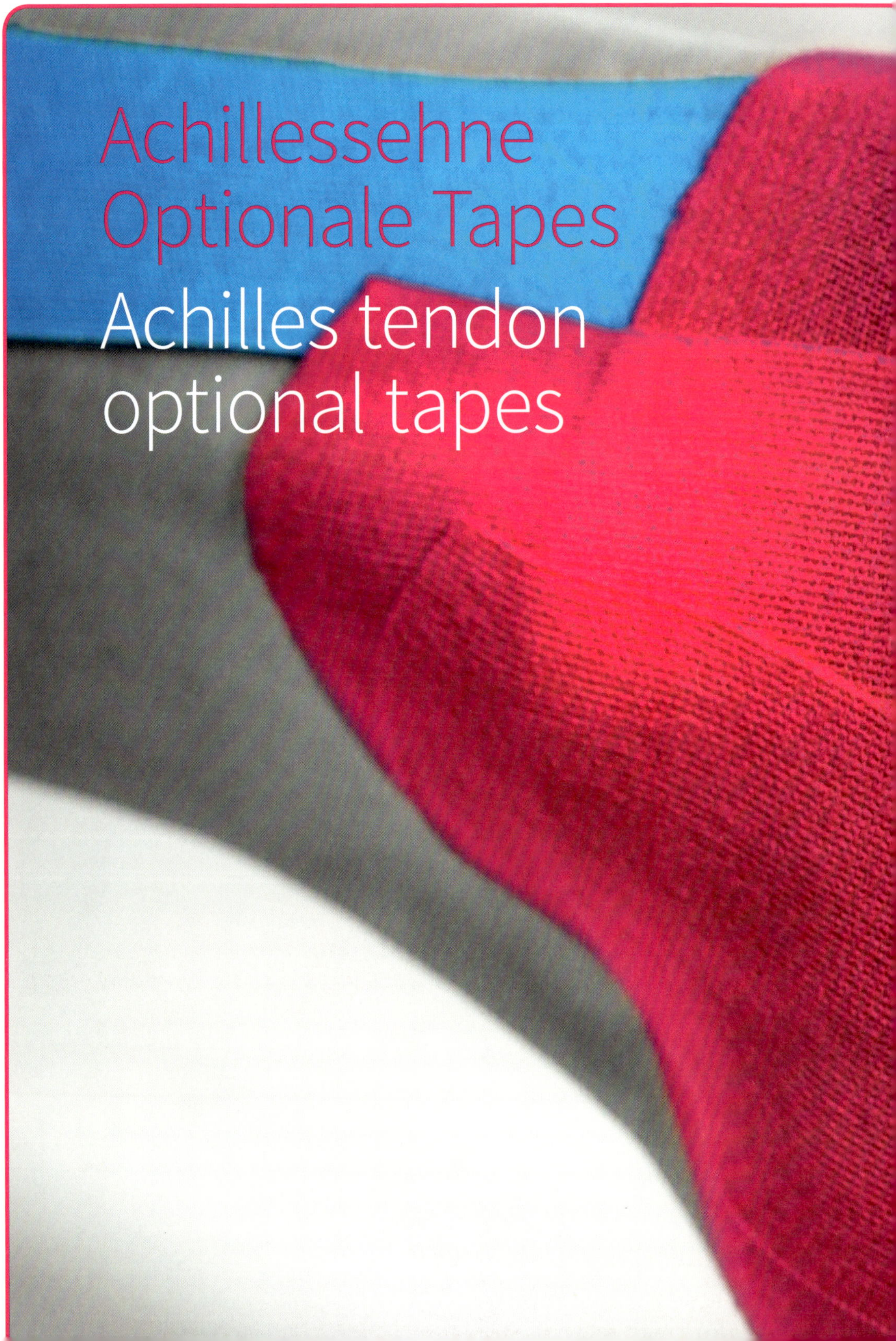

Achillessehne Optionale Tapes

Achilles tendon optional tapes

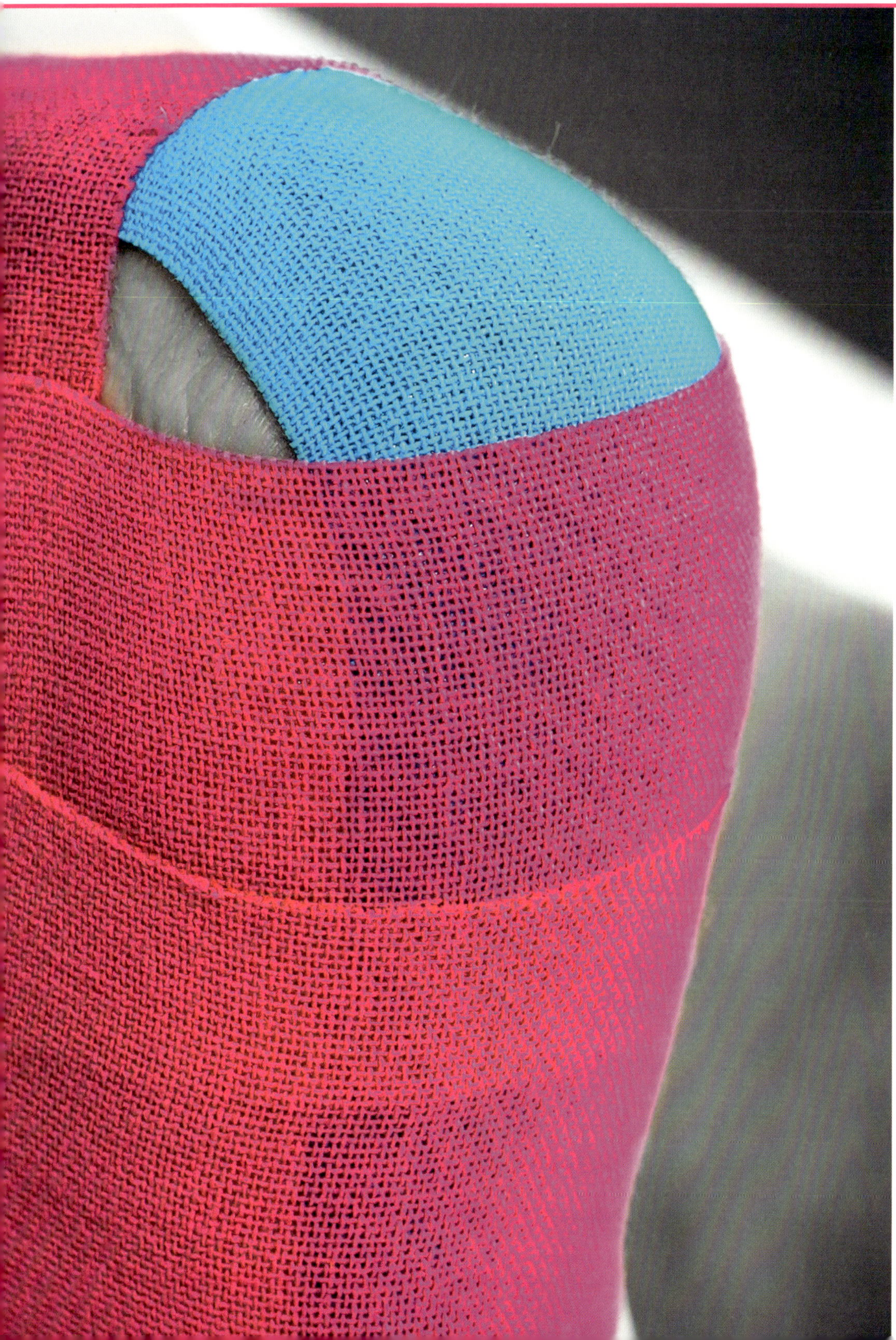

Achillessehne – Optionale Tapes
Achilles tendon – optional tapes

Bei starken Schmerzen am Sehnenansatz
For severe pain on tendon

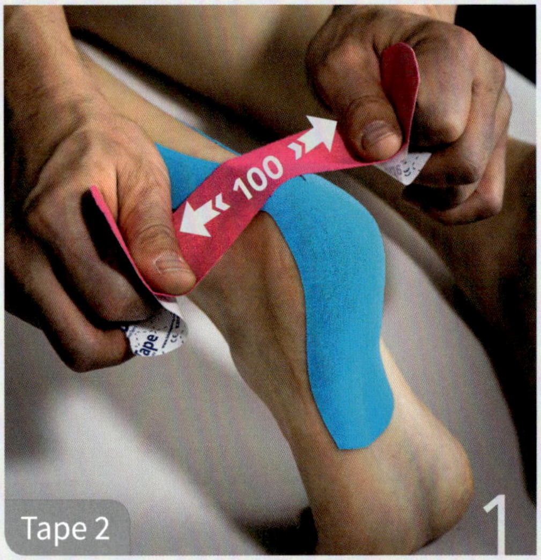

Ligamenttechnik

Ligament technique

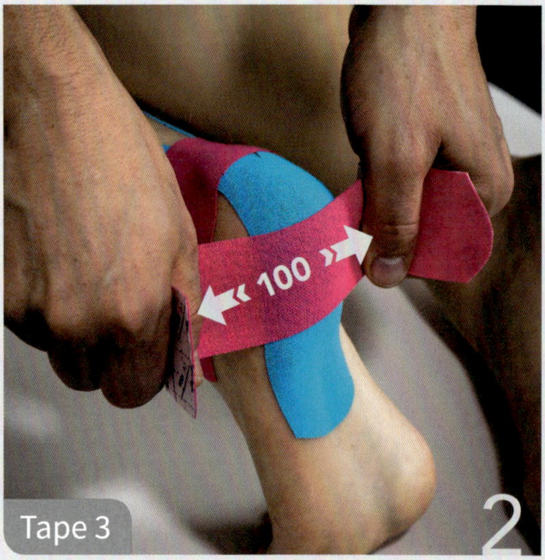

Ligamenttechnik

Ligament technique

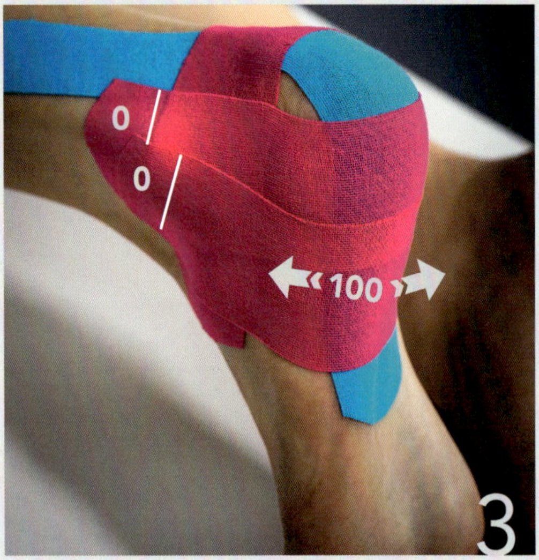

Fertig!

That's it!

Bitte nutzen Sie die Gitterpflaster zur Wirkungsverbesserung vor jeder Anwendung. Einfach auf die Schmerzpunkte kleben

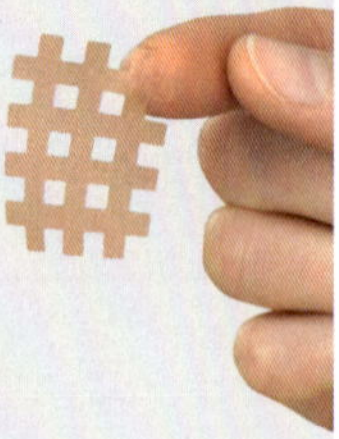

Please use the cross-tapes to improve the effect prior to each application Simply affix to the painful spots

Unsere Anwendungsbücher zu den Gitterpflastern ...

Our user manuals for lattice tape ...

Alle Bücher erhalten Sie auf www.okamed.de oder bei Amazon.

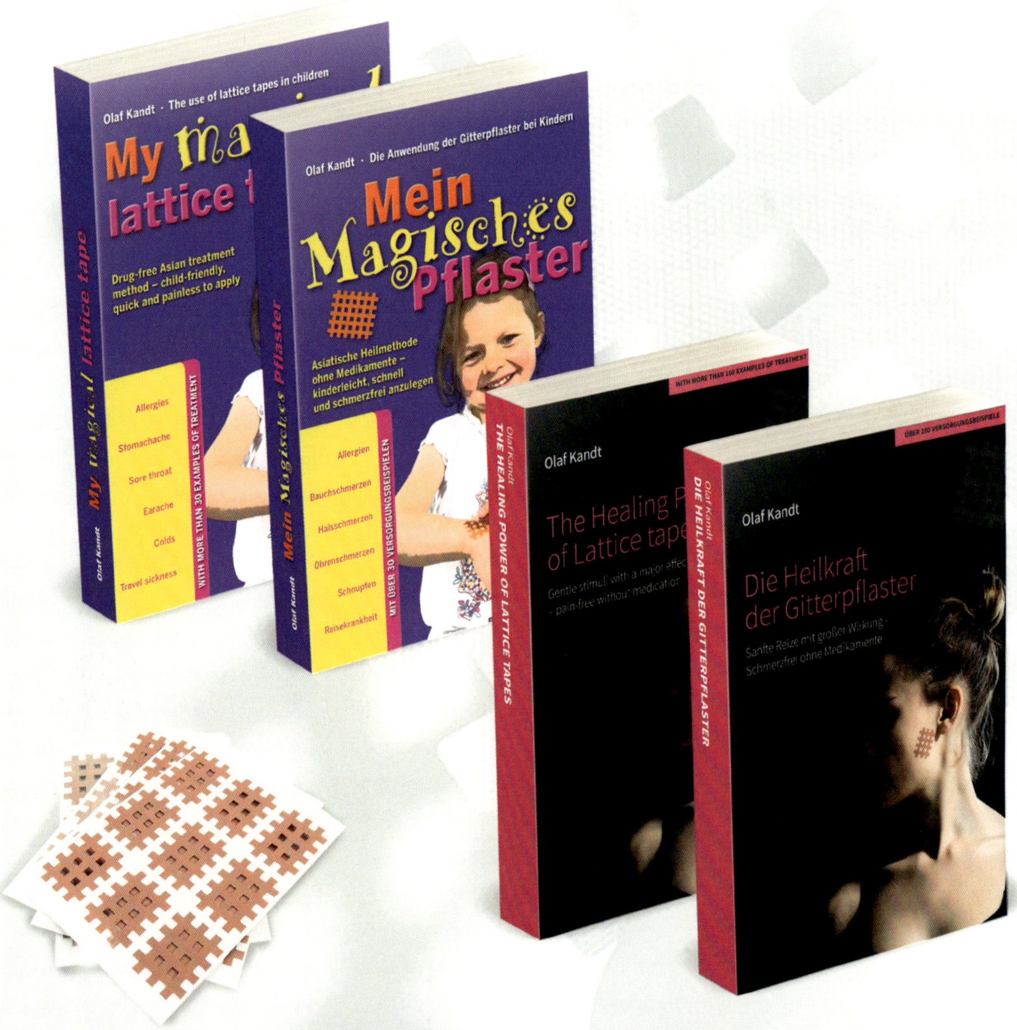

… und zum elastischen, kinesiologischen Tapen

… and our user manuals for elastic, kinesiology taping

All books available at www.okamed.com or at Amazon.

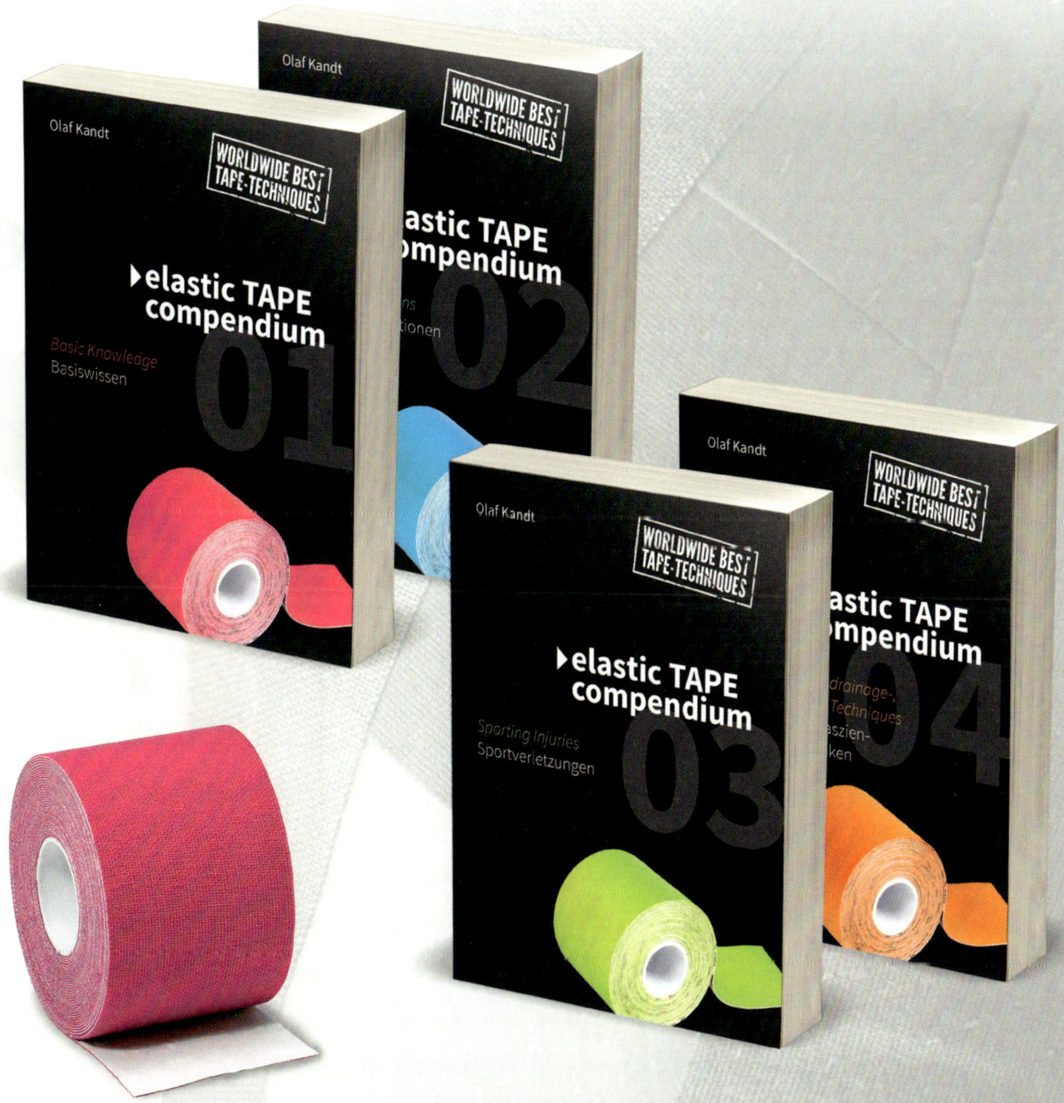

Anwendungsvideos mit und von Olaf Kandt

Auf www.okamed.de können Sie unsere Videos ansehen.

- Sie bekommen bei uns einen Zugang und haben vollen Zugriff auf alle Anwendungs-Videos.

User videos with and from Olaf Kandt

All our videos are available at www.okamed.com.

- You get access to the videos to watch them all.

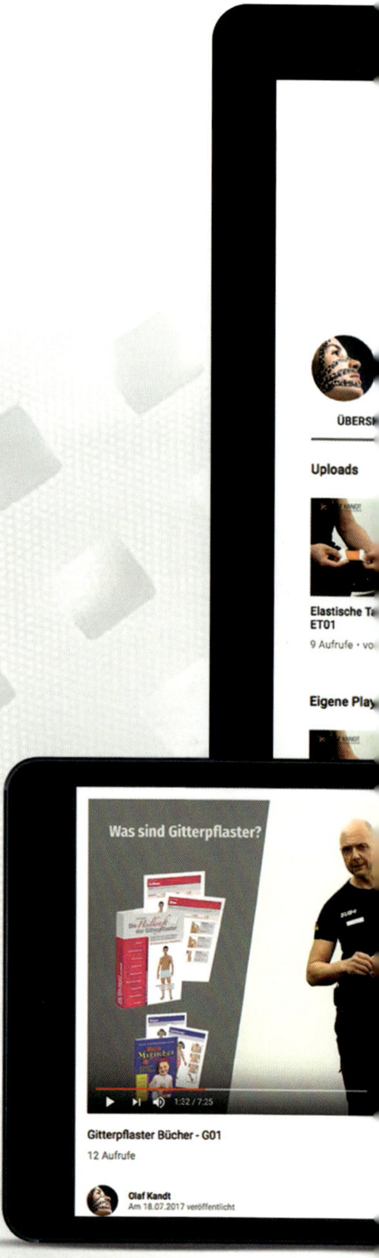

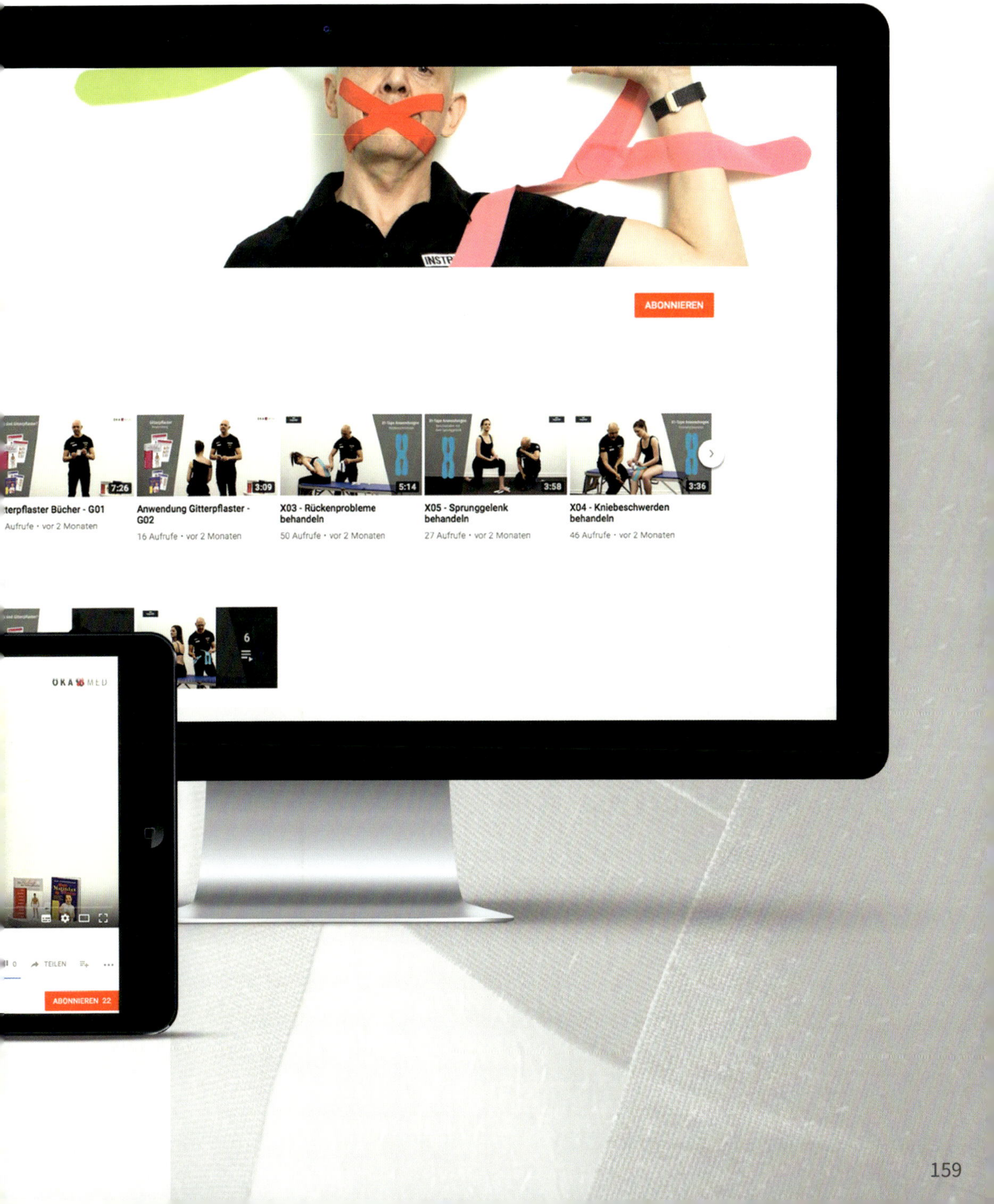
ABONNIEREN
terpflaster Bücher - G01
Aufrufe · vor 2 Monaten
Anwendung Gitterpflaster - G02
16 Aufrufe · vor 2 Monaten
X03 - Rückenprobleme behandeln
50 Aufrufe · vor 2 Monaten
X05 - Sprunggelenk behandeln
27 Aufrufe · vor 2 Monaten
X04 - Kniebeschwerden behandeln
46 Aufrufe · vor 2 Monaten
TEILEN
ABONNIEREN 22

Impressum

Olaf Kandt:
Elastic Tape Compendium
01-Basiswissen
Dezember 2017

1. Auflage
ISBN 978-3-9819380-1-2
Gedruckt in Deutschland

Autor und Verlag
Olaf Kandt
Hasloher Weg 1e
D-25474 Bönningstedt

www.okamed.de

Der Autor haftet nicht für etwaige Schäden, welche durch die Anwendung wie im Buch beschrieben, entstanden sind.

Druck
Eurodruck Hamburg
www.eurodruck.org

Design, Kreation und Produktion
inhouse – Print & Production
www.inhouse-print.de

ayeQ-benu GmbH
www.ayeQ-benu.com

Bilder
Okamed
Photography Schaarschmidt
Ulrich Schaarschmidt
fotolia

Verwendete Materialien
BB Tape:
WeTAPE Inc. / ALTERMED CO., LTD – Seoul, Korea

Gitterpflaster:
ATEX CO., LTD – Seoul, Korea

Ähnliche Produkte anderer Hersteller können jederzeit für die Anwendungen eingesetzt werden.

Legal notices

Olaf Kandt:
Elastic Tape Compendium
01-Basic Knowledge
December 2017

1st edition
ISBN 978-3-9819380-1-2
Printed in Germany

Author and publisher
Olaf Kandt
Hasloher Weg 1e
D-25474 Bönningstedt

www.okamed.com

The author accepts no liability for any injuries which occur due to use as described in the book.

Printer
Eurodruck Hamburg
www.eurodruck.org

Design, creation and production
inhouse – Print & Production
www.inhouse-print.de

ayeQ-benu GmbH
www.ayeQ-benu.com

Pictures
Okamed
Photography Schaarschmidt
Ulrich Schaarschmidt
fotolia

Used materials
BB Tape:
WeTAPE Inc. / ALTERMED CO., LTD – Seoul, Korea

Cross-tapes:
ATEX CO., LTD – Seoul, Korea

Similar products from different suppliers can be used for application at any time.